Clinical Practice Guideline

Number 9

Management of Cancer Pain

Management of Cancer Pain Guideline Panel

Ada Jacox, RN, PhD (Co-Chair)
Daniel B. Carr, MD (Co-Chair)
Richard Payne, MD (Co-Chair)
Charles B. Berde, MD, PhD
William Brietbart, MD
Joanna M. Cain, MD
C. Richard Chapman, PhD
Charles S. Cleeland, PhD
Betty R. Ferrell, RN, PhD
Rebecca S. Finley, PharmD, MS
Nancy O. Hester, RN, PhD
C. Stratton Hill, Jr., MD
W. David Leak, MD
Arthur G. Lipman, PharmD
Catherine L. Logan
Charles L. McGarvey, PT, MS
Christine A. Miaskowski, RN, PhD
David Stevenson Mulder, MD
Judith A. Paice, RN, PhD
Barbara S. Shapiro, MD
Edward B. Silberstein, MD
Rev. Robert S. Smith, PhD
Jeanne Stover
Carole V. Tsou, MD
Loretta Vecchiarelli
David E. Weissman, MD

U.S. Department of Health and Human Services
Public Health Service
Agency for Health Care Policy and Research

AHCPR Publication No. 94-0592
March 1994

Guideline Development and Use

Guidelines are systematically developed statements to assist practitioner and patient decisions about appropriate health care for specific clinical conditions. This guideline was developed by a multidisciplinary panel of private-sector clinicians and other experts convened by the Agency for Health Care Policy and Research (AHCPR). The panel employed an explicit, science-based methodology and expert clinical judgment to develop specific statements on patient assessment and management for the clinical condition selected.

Extensive literature searches were conducted, and critical reviews and syntheses were used to evaluate empirical evidence and significant outcomes. Peer review and field review were undertaken to evaluate the validity, reliability, and utility of the guideline in clinical practice. The panel's recommendations are primarily based on the published scientific literature. When the scientific literature was incomplete or inconsistent in a particular area, the recommendations reflect the professional judgment of panel members and consultants. In some instances, there was not unanimity of opinion.

The guideline reflects the state of knowledge, current at the time of publication, on effective and appropriate care. Given the inevitable changes in the state of scientific information and technology, periodic review, updating, and revision will be done. We believe that the AHCPR-assisted clinical guideline development process will make positive contributions to the quality of care in the United States. We encourage practitioners and patients to use the information provided in this clinical practice guideline. The recommendations may not be appropriate for use in all circumstances. Decisions to adopt any particular recommendation must be made by the practitioner in light of available resources and circumstances presented by individual patients.

J. Jarrett Clinton, MD
Administrator
Agency for Health Care Policy and Research

Publication of this guideline does not necessarily represent endorsement by the U.S. Department of Health and Human Services.

Foreword

Cancer is increasingly prevalent in the United States, and the pain associated with it is frequently undertreated. Cancer is diagnosed in over one million Americans annually, and one of five deaths in the United States—about 1,400 per day—results from cancer.

Patients with cancer often have multiple pain problems, but in most patients, the pain can be effectively controlled. Nevertheless, undertreatment is common because of a lack of knowledge by clinicians about effective assessment and management, negative attitudes of patients and clinicians toward the use of drugs for pain relief, and a variety of problems related to drug regulations, and the cost of and reimbursement for effective pain management.

This guideline was developed by an interdisciplinary panel of clinicians, patients, researchers, and experts in health policy. The guideline provides a synthesis of scientific research and expert judgment to make recommendations on pain assessment and management. Approximately 470 health care professionals and 70 patients were involved either as consultants and peer reviewers or as participants in pilot testing.

The *Clinical Practice Guideline for the Management of Cancer Pain* was commissioned by the Agency for Health Care Policy and Research (AHCPR). It follows and makes reference to an earlier guideline on acute pain management after surgery or trauma, also commissioned by AHCPR. The cancer pain guideline includes a section on the management of HIV positive/AIDS-related pain because of similarities in the sources of pain and the management approaches. This guideline is designed to help clinicians understand the assessment and treatment of cancer pain and associated symptoms. It reflects a multimodal approach to the management of pain, and it emphasizes the need for careful and continuous assessment to match interventions to the sources of pain in individual patients.

Abstract

Cancer is diagnosed in over one million Americans annually, and one of five deaths in the United States—about 1,400 per day—result from cancer. Despite recent advances in the understanding of pain and pain management approaches, pain control remains a significant problem for patients with cancer. This guideline is designed to help any clinician who works with any oncology patient in any setting to understand the assessment and treatment of pain and associated symptoms.

The guideline was developed by an interdisciplinary panel of clinicians, patients, and experts in health policy. The panel used a combination of scientific evidence and expert judgment to make recommendations about pain management in patients with cancer.

The guideline makes recommendations about the assessment and management of pain. Interventions described include the use of (1) analgesics and adjuvant drugs; (2) cognitive/behavior strategies; (3) physical modalities; (4) palliative radiation and antineoplastic therapies; (5) nerve blocks; and (6) palliative and ablative surgery.

The cost of cancer pain in suffering, disability, and quality of life is high. The guidelines recommend that cancer pain be treated aggressively by pharmacologic and nonpharmacologic approaches. In most instances, pain can be treated effectively with relatively low-cost, noninvasive therapies. Given this evidence, health system barriers that interfere with effective pain management—such as restrictive legislation regarding the uses of opioid analgesics and third-party payer practices that do not reimburse for less invasive interventions—should be changed.

Jacox A, Carr DB, Payne R, et al. *Management of Cancer Pain. Clinical Practice Guideline* No. 9. AHCPR Publication No. 94-0592. Rockville, MD. Agency for Health Care Policy and Research, U.S. Department of Health and Human Services, Public Health Service, March 1994.

Dedication

The *Clinical Practice Guideline for the Management of Cancer Pain* is dedicated to the memory of Jeanne Stover, a member of the panel that developed the guidelines. Jeanne represented the National Coalition for Cancer Survivorship on the panel. A 23-year survivor of breast cancer, she had metastatic disease during the last 9 years of her life and succumbed to this disease during her tenure as a panel member. She was a founding member of Living Through Cancer, a cancer self-help group in Albuquerque, New Mexico. The panel appreciates the insights and wisdom that Jeanne shared with us.

Panel Members

Ada Jacox, RN, PhD, FAAN,   **(1991–94)**
Co-Chair
Independence Foundation Chair in Health Policy
School of Nursing
The Johns Hopkins University
Baltimore, Maryland
Specialties: Health Policy, Outcomes Research

Daniel B. Carr, MD, Co-Chair,   **(1991–92)**
Special Consultant (1992–94)
Director, Division of Pain Management
Department of Anesthesia
Massachusetts General Hospital
Boston, Massachusetts
Specialties: Anesthesiology, Endocrinology

Richard Payne, MD, Member   **(1991–94)**
Co-Chair (1992–94)
Director, Pain and Symptom Management Section
MD Anderson Cancer Center
Houston, Texas
Specialties: Neurology, Oncology

Charles B. Berde, MD, PhD   **(1992–94)**
Director, Pain Treatment Service
Children's Hospital
Boston, Massachusetts
Specialties: Pediatrics, Anesthesia, Critical Care

William Breitbart, MD   **(1991–94)**
Associate Member
Memorial Sloan-Kettering Cancer Center
New York, New York
Specialty: Psychiatry, Internal Medicine

Joanna M. Cain, MD   **(1992–94)**
Director, Women's Clinic
Division of Gynecologic Oncology
University of Washington Hospital
Seattle, Washington
Specialties: Obstetrics, Gynecologic Oncology

C. Richard Chapman, PhD   (1991–92)
Professor, Department of Anesthesiology
University of Washington School of Medicine
Director, Pain and Toxicity Research Program
Fred Hutchinson Cancer Research Center
Seattle, Washington
Specialty: Psychology

Charles S. Cleeland, PhD   (1992–94)
Director, Pain Research Group
Professor, Neurology
Department of Neurology
University of Wisconsin Medical School
Madison, Wisconsin
Specialty: Psychology

Betty R. Ferrell, RN, PhD, FAAN   (1991–94)
Associate Research Scientist, Nursing Research
City of Hope Medical Center
Duarte, California
Specialties: Oncology, Nursing

Rebecca S. Finley, PharmD, MS   (1992–94)
Head, Section of Pharmacy Services
University of Maryland Cancer Center
Associate Professor of Oncology
Associate Professor of Pharmacy Practice
University of Maryland School of Pharmacy
Baltimore, Maryland
Specialty: Institutional Pharmacy

Nancy O. Hester, RN, PhD, FAAN   (1991–94)
Associate Professor, School of Nursing
University of Colorado Health Sciences Center
Denver, Colorado
Specialties: Pediatrics, Research Methods

C. Stratton Hill, Jr., MD   (1991–92)
Professor of Medicine
University of Texas
MD Anderson Cancer Center
Houston, Texas
Specialty: Oncology

W. David Leak, MD, FACPM (1992–94)
Medical Director, Pain Control Consultants
Adjunct Staff, Cleveland Clinic Foundation
Westerville, Ohio
Specialty: Pain Medicine

Arthur G. Lipman, PharmD (1991–92)
Professor of Clinical Pharmacy
College of Pharmacy
University of Utah
Salt Lake City, Utah
Specialty: Pharmacology in Pain Symptom Control

Catherine L. Logan (1992–94)
Executive Director and Founder, Living Through Cancer, Inc.
Board of Advisors, National Coalition for Cancer Survivorship
Albuquerque, New Mexico
Consumer Representative

Charles L. McGarvey, PT, MS (1991–92)
Chief, Physical Therapy Section
Rehabilitation Medicine Department
Warren G. Magnuson Clinical Center
National Institutes of Health
Bethesda, Maryland
Specialty: Physical Therapy

Christine A. Miaskowski, RN, PhD, FAAN (1991–92)
Associate Professor, Department of Physiological Nursing
University of California, San Francisco
San Francisco, California
Specialty: Oncology

David Stevenson Mulder, MD (1991–92)
Professor of Surgery, McGill University
Surgeon-in-Chief, Montreal General Hospital
Montreal, Quebec, Canada
Specialty: Cardiothoracic Surgery

Judith A. Paice, RN, PhD (1992–94)
Clinical Specialist, Pain Management
Neuroscience Institute
Rush-Presbyterian-St. Luke's Medical Center
Chicago, Illinois
Specialty: Neurosurgery, Oncology

Barbara S. Shapiro, MD (1991–92)
Associate Director, Pain Management Program
Children's Hospital of Philadelphia
Assistant Professor of Pediatrics
University of Pennsylvania School of Medicine
Philadelphia, Pennsylvania
Specialties: General Pediatrics, Pain Management

Edward B. Silberstein, MD, FACNP (1992–94)
Associate Director, E. L. Saenger Radioisotope Laboratory
University of Cincinnati Medical Center
Professor of Medicine and Radiology
University of Cincinnati College of Medicine
Cincinnati, Ohio
Specialties: Nuclear Medicine, Internal Medicine,
Hematology, Oncology

Rev. Robert S. Smith, PhD (1991–92)
Director, Institute for Medicine in Contemporary Society
State University Medical Center at Stony Brook
Stony Brook, New York
Specialty: Religion, Ethics

Jeanne Stover (1991–92)
Cofounder of Living Through Cancer, Inc.
Sandia Park, New Mexico
Consumer Representative

Carole V. Tsou, MD (1991–92)
Residency Program Director
University of Hawaii
Department of Family Practice
Mililani, Hawaii
Specialty: Family Medicine

Loretta Vecchiarelli (1991–92)
Rehabilitation Hospital of Western New England
Ludlow, Massachusetts
Consumer Representative

David E. Weissman, MD (1992–94)
Associate Professor of Medicine
Division of Cancer and Blood Diseases
Medical College of Wisconsin
Milwaukee, Wisconsin
Specialties: Internal Medicine, Oncology

Acknowledgments

The Cancer Pain Management Panel expresses profound appreciation to the patients who helped us in the development of the consumer version of the guideline and to our numerous colleagues in many disciplines who made valuable contributions during the development of the guideline. The scientific reviewers critiqued sections or complete drafts of the guideline document, and a variety of individuals pilot tested the guideline. A full listing of those involved in this effort appears in the list of contributors at the end of the document. Special recognition goes to Ehud Arbit, MD, Andrew Brown, MB BS, Stuart DuPen, MD, Nora Janjan, MD, Mathew Lefkowitz, MD, Margo McCaffery, RN, MS, Raphael Pollock, MD, PhD, Karen Syjala, PhD, Anna Williams, RN, MN, and Melissa Wolff, RT, MS—all of whom provided original text for the document. We also acknowledge the extraordinary review efforts of Charles Coté, MD, June Dahl, PhD, Stuart Grossman, MD, Philipp Lippe, MD, Margo McCaffery, RN, MS, Patricia McGrath, PhD, Richard Patt, MD, Vivian Sheidler, RN, MS, Thomas Smith, MD, and Sridhar Vasudevan, MD. These individuals provided major and repeated reviews of various aspects of the guideline, as well as valuable advice to the panel chairs.

We acknowledge the critical approach and tireless, energetic efforts to the many aspects of guideline development of Jane Ballantyne, MB, Elon Eisenberg, MD, Donna Mahrenholz, RN, PhD, and particularly Janice Ulmer, RN, PhD, all of whom served as staff to the panel. Dr. Patricia Stephens provided excellent and timely editing for several drafts of the guideline. Research assistants who provided valuable services in reviewing the literature included Dorothy Herron, RN, MSN, Yeonghee Shin, RN, PhD, and Joyce Willens, RN, MSN. Other valuable services in the preparation of various materials were provided by research assistants Leslie Dunham, Stella Seal, Sabreena Woods, and our secretary, Yvonne Deane-Hibbert, at the Johns Hopkins University. Drs. Frederick Mosteller, Thomas Chalmers, and Catherine Berkey of the Technology Assessment Group, Harvard School of Public Health, gave valuable guidance during literature reviews for meta-analyses. Miss Evelyn Hall, at Massachusetts General Hospital, provided expert secretarial assistance in the development of guideline materials. Drs. Richard Kitz and George Battit of the Massachusetts General Hospital provided ongoing support and encouragement for work at that site.

Contents

Executive Summary...1
1. Overview 7
    Scope of the Problem..7
    Importance of Controlling Cancer Pain 8
    Suffering, Loss of Control, and Quality of Life....................9
    Overview of Pain and Pain Management Modalities 11
    Barriers to Effective Pain Management 16
        Legal Regulation of Opioids 16
        Cost and Reimbursement for Pain Management 19
    Methods Used To Develop the Guideline........................20
    Organization of Guideline 21

2. Assessment of Pain in the Patient With Cancer..................23
    Initial Pain Assessment 24
    Ongoing Pain Assessment 28
    Assessment of Common Cancer Pain Syndromes................29
        Bone Metastases...30
        Epidural Metastases/Spinal Cord Compression 30
        Metastases to the Skull 31
        Plexopathies 31
        Peripheral Neuropathies 33
        Acute and Postherpetic Neuralgia 36
        Abdominal Pain 36
        Mucositis..37
    Assessment of New Pain 38

3. Pharmacologic Management.......................................39
    The WHO Ladder..41
    Nonsteroidal Anti-Inflammatory Drugs (NSAIDs).............46
    Opioids 49
        Tolerance and Physical Dependence........................50
        Dosage Titration..51
        Administration Methods 55
            Oral 55
            Rectal 56
            Transdermal...56
            Nasal 56
            Intravenous or Subcutaneous...............................57
            Intraspinal..57
            Intraventricular 59
            Patient-Controlled Analgesia (PCA) 59

Management of Side Effects 61
  Constipation 61
  Sedation...61
  Nausea and Vomiting 63
  Respiratory Depression....................................63
  Other Side Effects 64
Adjuvant Drugs...65
  Corticosteroids 65
  Anticonvulsants 65
  Antidepressants 67
  Neuroleptic Agents.......................................68
  Hydroxyzine 68
  Bisphosphonates and Calcitonin 69
  Placebos 69
Antineoplastic Therapies 70
Influence of Concurrent Medical Conditions
on Pharmacotherapy.......................................70
Pharmacologic Treatments Not Recommended..................71
Discharge Planning Regarding Medications....................71

**4. Nonpharmacologic Management: Physical and
Psychosocial Modalities.....................................75**
Introduction 76
Physical Modalities..76
  Cutaneous Stimulation 76
  Exercise...78
  Counterstimulation.......................................79
    TENS...79
    Acupuncture 79
Psychosocial Interventions..................................80
  Relaxation and Imagery...................................81
  Distraction and Reframing.................................82
  Patient Education 83
  Psychotherapy and Structured Support......................86
  Hypnosis...86
  Peer Support Groups......................................86
  Pastoral Counseling 87

5. Nonpharmacologic Interventions: Invasive Therapies 89
Introduction 90
Radiation Therapy 90
  Bone Metastases..91
    Pain Relief With Localized Radiation Therapy...........92
    Wide-Field Radiation Therapy 92
    Radiopharmaceuticals 93

Plexopathy..93
Other Therapeutic Applications 94
Brachytherapy..94
Anesthetic Techniques..95
Nerve Blocks 95
Catheter Placement for Drug Delivery 98
Neurosurgery...99
Neuroablation...100
Peripheral Neurectomy....................................100
Dorsal Rhizotomy 100
Anterolateral Cordotomy (Spinal Tractotomy).........100
Commissural Myelotomy 101
Hypophysectomy 101
Neuraxial Opioid Infusion 102
Neuroaugmentation 102
Surgery 103
Surgical Management of Pain Due to Primary or
Metastatic Tumor...103
Pain as a Consequence of Operation 105

6. **Procedure-Related Pain in Adults and Children** 107
Managing Procedure-Related Pain..............................108
Pharmacologic Strategies for Procedural Pain 108
Sedation for Procedural Pain. 112
Additional Pain Management Strategies for
Lumbar Puncture and Bone Marrow Aspiration 113

7. **Pain in Special Populations**......................................115
Pain in Neonates, Children, and Adolescents....................116
Assessment 117
Methods for Assessing Pain...................................118
Self-Report 118
Behavioral Observation 119
Pain Management 120
Medical Interventions 120
Analgesics and Adjuvants................................120
Analgesics for Neonates and Young Infants 124
Epidural Analgesia 126
Nonpharmacologic Methods 126
Assessing the Adequacy of Pain Management Strategies...127
Elderly Patients 127
Patients With Psychiatric Problems Associated
With Cancer Pain 130
Depression in Patients With Cancer Pain....................131
Suicide and Cancer Pain 132

Anxiety 133
Delirium and Its Effects on Treating Pain 134
Substance Abusers 134
Minority Populations 138
Pain in Patients With AIDS 139

8. Monitoring the Quality of Pain Management 143

References 147

Acronyms 183

Glossary 185

Contributors 189

Attachment A 219

Attachment B 227

Attachment C 241

Index 247

Tables

1. Effect of cancer pain on quality of life 11
2. Barriers to cancer pain management 17
3. Initial pain assessment 25
4. Metastases to the skull 32
5. Common cancer pain syndromes due to peripheral nerve injury 34
6. Common causes of abdominal pain 36
7. Assessment of mucositis 37
8. Advantages and disadvantages of pain therapies 42
9. Dosing data for acetaminophen (APAP) and NSAIDs 48
10. Dose equivalents for opioid analgesics for opioid-naive adults and children ≥50 kg body weight 52
11. Dose equivalents for opioid analgesics for opioid-naive children and adults <50 kg body weight 54
12. Intraspinal drug delivery systems 60
13. General comments and cautions regarding the use of opioid analgesics 62
14. Adjuvant analgesic drugs for cancer pain 66
15. Drugs and routes of administration not recommended for long-term treatment of cancer pain 72

16. Patient education program content 84
17. Sources of information for patients and their families........85
18. How to find local support groups 87
19. Nerve blocks...95
20. General principles of management for
    painful procedures 109
21. Pharmacologic agents for management of
    procedural pain...111
22. Checklist for assessing adequacy of pain management
    in children 128
23. Risk factors that predispose cancer patient to
    depressive disorders......................................132
24. Suicide risk factors in cancer patients with pain.............133

Figures
1. Flowchart: continuing pain management in patients
   with cancer...13
2. The WHO three-step analgesic ladder........................14
3. Pain management strategies: a hierarchy 15
4. Pain intensity scales 26
5. Pain management plan 74

Executive Summary

Pain control in people with cancer remains a significant problem in health care even though cancer pain can be managed effectively in up to 90 percent of patients. Recognition of the widespread undertreatment of cancer pain has prompted recent corrective efforts from health care disciplines, professional and consumer organizations, and governments throughout the world.

The *Clinical Practice Guideline for the Management of Cancer Pain* was commissioned by the Agency for Health Care Policy and Research (AHCPR). It follows and makes reference to a 1992 guideline on acute pain management after surgery or trauma, also commissioned by AHCPR. This guideline is designed to help clinicians who work with oncology patients to understand the assessment and treatment of pain and associated symptoms. It also discusses briefly the management of pain in patients with human immunodeficiency virus (HIV) and/or acquired immunodeficiency syndrome (AIDS).

The guideline has ten goals:

■ To inform clinicians and patients and their families that most cancer pain can be relieved by available methods.

■ To dispel unfounded fears that addiction results from the appropriate use of medications to control cancer pain.

■ To inform clinicians that cancer pain:

Accompanies both disease and treatment.

Changes over time.

May have multiple simultaneous causes.

If unrelieved, can affect the physical, psychological, social, and spiritual well-being of the patient.

■ To promote prompt and effective assessment, diagnosis, and treatment of pain in patients with cancer.

■ To strengthen the ability of patients with cancer and their families to communicate new or unrelieved pain in order to secure prompt evaluation and effective treatment.

■ To provide clinicians with a synthesis of the literature and expert opinion for application to the management of cancer pain.

■ To familiarize patients and their families with options available for pain relief and to promote their active participation in selecting among these.

- To provide a model for cancer pain management to guide therapy in selected painful, life-threatening conditions such as AIDS.

- To provide information and guidelines on the use of controlled substances for the treatment of cancer pain that distinguish the use of these drugs for legitimate medical purposes from their abuse as illegitimate drugs.

- To identify health policy and research issues that affect cancer pain management.

Not all cancer pain or associated symptoms can be entirely eliminated, but available approaches, when appropriately and attentively applied, effectively relieve pain in most patients. The importance of effective pain management extends beyond analgesia to encompass the patient's quality of life and ability to function in the family and society.

Because patients vary greatly in their diagnoses and stage of disease progression, their responses to pain and interventions, and their personal preferences, the guideline offers a flexible approach to the management of cancer pain that clinicians can use in daily practice and adapt, as appropriate, to the treatment of painful noncancerous conditions.

The guideline emphasizes:

- A collaborative, interdisciplinary approach to pain control, including all members of the health care team, with participation of the patient and the patient's family.

- An individualized pain control plan developed and agreed on by patients, their families, and practitioners.

- Ongoing assessment of the patient's pain.

- Both drug and nondrug therapies to prevent and/or control pain.

- A formalized, institutional approach to the management of cancer pain, with clear lines of responsibility for pain management and for monitoring the quality of pain management.

The guideline includes general strategies for pain management, as well as the management of specific pain syndromes, and it addresses issues related to special populations. It also contains a pain management flowchart, analgesic dosage tables, sample pain assessment tools, examples of nondrug interventions, and information about resources for patients and their families.

The first chapter is an overview of the prevalence of cancer and cancer pain. A key recommendation is that clinicians should reassure patients and their families that most pain can be relieved safely and effectively. Barriers to effective cancer pain management identified by the panel include problems related to health care professionals, to patients, and to the health care and drug regulatory system. The panel recommends that curricula for health professionals include sufficient content on pain to prepare clinicians to assess and manage pain effectively. The panel acknowledges that clinicians need to educate patients and their families about pain and its management and to encourage patients to be active participants in their care. Clinicians are encouraged to collaborate with patients and families, taking costs of drugs and technologies into account in selecting pain management strategies. The panel noted the need for Federal, State, and local laws and regulatory policies to be developed so as not to hamper the appropriate use of opioid analgesics for cancer pain. The first chapter presents a flowchart that indicates the need to use multiple modalities concurrently in pain management and emphasizes the need to begin with the least invasive methods capable of controlling the pain, titrating the pain treatment to the patient's needs. The process whereby panelists were selected, the methods used in the development of the guideline, and a summary of the scientific evidence for the interventions are presented.

Chapter 2 emphasizes the need for health professionals to ask patients about pain and to accept the patient's self-report as the primary source of assessment. The need for comprehensive assessment and careful documentation is discussed, with attention to initial evaluation and appraisal of any new pain that emerges. A mnemonic for the recommended clinical approach is given.

A discussion of the assessment of common cancer pain syndromes includes bone metastases, epidural metastases/spinal cord compression, plexopathies, peripheral neuropathies, acute and postherpetic neuralgia, abdominal pain, and mucositis.

The pharmacologic management of pain is presented in Chapter 3. The importance of individualizing the regimen to the patient and of using the simplest dosage schedules and least invasive pain management modalities is emphasized. The World Health Organization's analgesic ladder is discussed, with suggestions about how various drugs should be used alone and in combination. The need to make a distinction between opioid tolerance and physical dependence on the one hand and "addiction" on the other is stressed because the pervasive misconception that these three entities are the same hinders effective pain management.

Chapter 3 describes the use of nonsteroidal anti-inflammatory drugs and opioids, and discusses how to titrate drugs to effect for individual patients. Various routes of administration and the management of drug side effects are discussed. The panel noted that respiratory depression is infrequently a significant limiting factor in pain management because,

3

with repeated doses, tolerance develops. This tolerance allows adequate pain treatment without much risk of respiratory compromise. The person dying from cancer should not be allowed to live out life with unrelieved pain because of a fear of side effects; rather, appropriate, aggressive, palliative support should be given. The use of adjuvant drugs to increase the analgesic efficacy of opioids, to treat concurrent symptoms that exacerbate pain, and to provide independent analgesia for specific types of pain is described. Careful discharge planning when a patient moves from one setting to another is emphasized.

Chapters 4 and 5 discuss the nonpharmacologic management of pain. Chapter 4 includes recommendations for the use of physical modalities, including the use of superficial heat and cold, massage, exercise, transcutaneous electrical nerve stimulation, and acupuncture, and psychosocial interventions, including relaxation and imagery, distraction and reframing, patient education, psychotherapy and structured support, and hypnosis. For each modality, brief explanations are given regarding the mechanisms of operation and practical ways in which they can be applied in the patient care setting. The importance of referring patients to peer support groups and providing pastoral counseling for those who wish it is also emphasized.

Chapter 5 discusses more invasive therapies, including palliative radiation, anesthetic techniques including nerve blocks, neurosurgery, and palliative surgery. The panel recommends that, with rare exception, noninvasive treatment should precede invasive palliative approaches.

Chapter 6 describes the management of procedure-related pain. It discusses the use of drugs and other approaches for the relief of pain produced by the multiple invasive procedures that patients undergo as part of their treatment.

The discussion thus far in the guideline is largely focused on adult patients. Chapter 7 includes a discussion of a number of special populations for whom clinicians should give special attention and considerations, including the very young and very old, the cognitively impaired, known or suspected substance abusers, and non-English-speaking persons. When developing a pain treatment plan, clinicians should be aware of the unique needs and circumstances of patients from various ethnic and cultural backgrounds. The need for assessment methods appropriate for neonates, children, and adolescents is stressed. Elderly patients should be considered at risk for undertreatment of pain. Uncontrolled pain is an important factor contributing to feelings of hopelessness, suicidal ideation, and requests for clinician-assisted suicide or euthanasia; therefore, it should be aggressively assessed and treated. Because patients with current substance abuse disorders are at risk for undertreatment of cancer pain, their care should be managed by clinicians knowledgeable in both pain management and substance abuse. Because patients with HIV positive/AIDS often have pain problems similar to those of patients with cancer, recommendations for pain assessment and management in this guideline generally should be used for pain in these patients.

Chapter 8 discusses the need for monitoring the quality of pain management and for developing formal means within each institution to evaluate pain management practices and to obtain patient feedback to gauge the adequacy of pain control. Institutional policy should define who is responsible for pain management, the acceptable level of patient monitoring, and the appropriate roles and limits of practice for health care providers.

The nearly 500 consultants, peer reviewers, and site reviewers who contributed to the development of the guideline are listed. The Attachments contain tables showing the strength of evidence for recommendations, pain assessment instruments, and sample relaxation exercises.

Explanation of Strength of Evidence

This guideline contains recommendations at the beginning of each chapter. Recommendations are followed in parentheses by a rating of the strength of evidence.

When the strength of evidence is A or B, the panel's recommendations are based primarily on the evidence. When the strength of recommendation is C or D, the panel used the available empirical evidence but based their recommendations primarily on expert judgment. When the recommendation is a statement of panel opinion regarding desirable practice and there is evidence that the practice is not commonly being followed, the term "panel consensus" is used.

A more complete explanation of strength of evidence is contained in Attachment A.

1 Overview

Recommendations

1. Clinicians should reassure patients and their families that most pain can be relieved safely and effectively. (A)

2. Clinicians should assess patients and, if pain is present, provide optimal relief throughout the course of illness. (Panel Consensus)

3. Curricula for health professionals should include sufficient content on pain to prepare clinicians to assess and manage pain effectively. (Panel Consensus)

4. Clinicians should include patient and family education about pain and its management in the treatment plan and encourage patients to be active participants in pain management. (A)

5. Federal, State, and local laws and regulatory polices should not hamper the appropriate use of opioid analgesics for cancer pain. (Panel Consensus)

6. Clinicians should collaborate with patients and families, taking costs of drugs and technologies into account in selecting pain management strategies. (Panel Consensus)

Scope of the Problem

Cancer is diagnosed in over 1 million Americans annually. About 8 million Americans now have cancer or a history of cancer; half of these diagnoses were made within the past 5 years. Cancer causes 1 of every 10 deaths worldwide (Stjernsward and Teoh, 1990) and is increasingly prevalent in the United States, where it causes 1 of 5 deaths--about 1,400 per day (American Cancer Society, 1994).

Pain associated with cancer is frequently undertreated in adults (Bonica, 1990) and children (Miser, Dothage, Wesley, et al., 1987). Patients with cancer often have multiple pain problems (Coyle, Adelhardt, Foley, et al., 1990). Cancer pain may be due to (1) tumor progression and related pathology (e.g., nerve damage), (2) operations and other invasive diagnostic or therapeutic procedures, (3) toxicities of chemotherapy and radiation, (4) infection, or (5) muscle aches when patients limit physical activity (Foley, 1979). The incidence of pain in patients with cancer depends on the type and stage of disease. At the time of diagnosis and at intermediate stages, 30 to 45 percent of patients experience moderate to severe pain

(Daut and Cleeland, 1982). On average, nearly 75 percent of patients with advanced cancer have pain. Of cancer patients with pain, 40 to 50 percent report it as moderate to severe, and another 25 to 30 percent describe it as very severe (Bonica, 1990).

In approximately 90 percent of patients, cancer pain can be controlled through relatively simple means (Goisis, Gorini, Ratti, et al., 1989; Schug, Zech, and Dörr, 1990; Teoh and Stjernsward, 1992; Ventafridda, Caraceni, and Gamba, 1990), yet a consensus statement from the National Cancer Institute Workshop on Cancer Pain indicated that the "undertreatment of pain and other symptoms of cancer is a serious and neglected public health problem" (National Cancer Institute, 1990). The Workshop concluded that "...every patient with cancer should have the expectation of pain control as an integral aspect of his/her care throughout the course of the disease" (National Cancer Institute, 1990).

Because cancer pain control is a problem of international scope, the World Health Organization (WHO) has urged that every nation give high priority to establishing a cancer pain relief policy (Stjernsward and Teoh, 1990). In the United States, many organizations have worked toward this goal (Ad Hoc Committee on Cancer Pain of the American Society of Clinical Oncology, 1992; American Pain Society, 1986; Health and Public Policy Committee, American College of Physicians, 1983; McGivney and Crooks, 1984; Spross, McGuire, and Schmitt, 1990a, 1990b, 1990c; Weissman, Burchman, Dinndorf, et al., 1988).

Importance of Controlling Cancer Pain

Pain control merits high priority for two reasons. First, unrelieved pain causes unnecessary suffering. Because pain diminishes activity, appetite, and sleep, it can further weaken already debilitated patients. The psychological effect of cancer pain can be devastating. Patients with cancer often lose hope when pain emerges, believing that pain heralds the inexorable progress of a feared, destructive, and fatal disease. Chronic unrelieved pain can lead patients to reject active treatment programs, and when their pain is severe or they are depressed, to consider or commit suicide. Besides mitigating suffering, pain control is important because, even when the underlying disease process is stable, uncontrolled pain prevents patients from working productively, enjoying recreation, or taking pleasure in their usual role in the family and society (Moinpour and Chapman, 1991). Pain control therefore merits a high priority not only for those with advanced disease, but also for the patient whose condition is stable and whose life expectancy is long.

Suffering, Loss of Control, and Quality of Life

A Patient's Perspective:

One of the worst aspects of cancer pain is that it's a constant reminder of the disease and of death. Many fear the pain will become unbearable before death, and those of us involved in support networks have seen these fears proven true.

Pain seems greater when dealing with it alone and an increasing number of us are finding comfort in support groups, where we also deal with issues of personal control, communication with doctors and nurses, effective adjunctive therapies, and other topics.

My dream is for a medication that can relieve my pain while leaving me alert and with no side effects.

—Jeanne Stover, Panel Member 1991–1992

Cancer pain may resolve with the patient's cure or continue indefinitely as a complication of otherwise curative therapy. Although cancer pain is often thought of as a crisis that emerges in advanced stages of disease, it may occur for many reasons and cause suffering, loss of control, and impaired quality of life throughout the patient's course of care, even for the patient whose condition is stable and whose life expectancy is long.

Suffering denotes an extended sense of threat to self-image and life, a perceived lack of options for coping with symptoms or problems caused by cancer, a sense of personal loss, and a lack of a basis for hope. "Suffering can include physical pain but is by no means limited to it.... Most generally, suffering can be defined as the state of severe distress associated with events that threaten the intactness of the person.... The suffering of patients with terminal cancer can often be relieved by demonstrating that their pain truly can be controlled" (Cassel, 1982).

Pain can exacerbate individual suffering by worsening helplessness, anxiety, and depression. Shock and disbelief, followed by symptoms of anxiety and depression (irritability and disruption of appetite and sleep, inability to concentrate or carry out usual activities) are common when people first learn they have cancer or discover that treatment has failed or disease has recurred (Massie and Holland, 1990). These symptoms usually resolve within a few weeks with support from family and caregivers, although medication to promote sleep and reduce anxiety may be necessary in crisis periods. "The relief of suffering and the cure of disease must be seen as twin obligations of a medical profession that is truly dedicated to the care of the sick" (Cassel, 1982).

> *The obligation to alleviate suffering is an essential component of the clinician's broader ethical duties to benefit and not harm; it dictates that health professionals maintain clinical expertise and knowledge in the management of pain, even when present educational programs do not provide this.*
>
> —*Cain and Hammes, in press; Hammes and Cain, in press*

Personal control refers to an individual's ability to shape immediate and long-range circumstances through one's own actions (Wallston, Wallston, Smith, et al., 1987), including:

■ Predicting events and outcomes successfully.

■ Exercising choice among options for action.

■ Maintaining a repertoire of coping skills.

■ Accessing and using relevant information.

■ Accessing and using social or other forms of support.

Personal control is undermined when cancer is diagnosed and is further reduced by ongoing pain, invasive or undignified procedures, treatment toxicities, hospitalization, and surgery. When pain reduces patients' options to exercise control, it diminishes psychological well-being and makes them feel helpless and vulnerable. Therefore, clinicians should support active patient involvement in effective and practical methods to manage pain.

The quality of life of cancer patients with pain is significantly worse than that of cancer patients without pain (Ferrell, Rhiner, Cohen, et al., 1991). Table 1 depicts the effect of pain in four quality-of-life domains—physical, psychological, spiritual, and social.

Family and loved ones of cancer patients share the suffering, loss of control, and impaired quality of life and also experience psychological and social stresses. Family caregivers need sleep and respite from the burdens of caregiving and may have socioeconomic needs and fears related to the costs of providing care.

Even in the absence of psychological, emotional, and physical stressors, the family may feel unprepared to deal with the patient's many needs. They often have to assess pain, make decisions about the amount and type of medication, and determine when the dose of medication is to be given. Sophisticated pain management strategies may require them to manage complex medication regimens involving parenteral or epidural infusions in the home.

Some family caregivers may hesitate to give adequate doses of pain medicines out of fear that the patient will become addicted or

Table 1. Effect of cancer pain on quality of life

Physical
    Decreased functional capability.
    Diminished strength, endurance.
    Nausea, poor appetite.
    Poor or interrupted sleep.

Psychological
    Diminished leisure, enjoyment.
    Increased anxiety, fear.
    Depression, personal distress.
    Difficulty concentrating.
    Somatic preoccupation.
    Loss of control.

Social
    Diminished social relationships.
    Decreased sexual function, affection.
    Altered appearance.
    Increased caregiver burden.

Spiritual
    Increased suffering.
    Altered meaning.
    Reevaluation of religious beliefs.

Source: Ferrell, Rhiner, Cohen, et al., 1991. Used with permission.

tolerant or develop respiratory depression (Ferrell, Cohen, Rhiner, et al., 1991). **Clinicians should reassure patients and families that most pain can be relieved safely and effectively.** Family caregivers may feel unprepared to deal with a patient's need for pain relief or may deny that the patient is in pain to avoid facing the possibility that the disease is progressing. These situations require ongoing discussions among patients, family caregivers, and experienced health care providers about pain management goals.

Overview of Pain and Pain Management Modalities

The anatomy, physiology, and pharmacology of pain and analgesia have been studied extensively. A major advance has been the finding that neural pathways that arise in the brain stem descend to the spinal cord and modulate activity in spinal nociceptive pathways (Fields and

Basbaum, 1978). These descending pathways, as well as related pain pathways within and above the spinal cord, respond to opioids and other analgesic drugs as well as physiologic and experimental stimuli, including stress (Mayer and Liebeskind, 1974), to produce analgesia. It has been speculated that the activation of this descending control system by the action of endogenous opioids such as β-endorphin and enkephalins may account for the phenomenon of placebo analgesia and the apparent analgesic effect of acupuncture in some clinical circumstances.

Pain may be defined as "an unpleasant sensory and emotional experience associated with actual or potential tissue damage, or described in terms of such damage" (International Association for the Study of Pain, Subcommittee on Taxonomy, 1979). Although the mechanisms of pain and pain pathways are becoming better understood, it should be emphasized that an individual's perception of pain and appreciation of its meaning are complex phenomena that involve psychological and emotional processes in addition to activation of nociceptive pathways (McGrath, 1990a). Pain intensity is not proportional to the type or extent of tissue damage but may be influenced at many sites within the nervous system. The perception of pain depends on the complex interactions between nociceptive and non-nociceptive impulses in ascending pathways, in relation to the activation of descending pain-inhibitory systems. This framework provides the basis for a comprehensive, multimodal approach to the assessment and treatment of patients with pain and fits with the clinical observation that there is no single approach to effective pain management. Instead, individualized pain management should take into account the stage of disease, concurrent medical conditions, characteristics of pain, and psychological and cultural characteristics of the patient. It also requires ongoing reassessment of the pain and treatment effectiveness.

Figure 1 is a flowchart depicting cancer pain management from the initial assessment of pain and its cause to the various treatment modalities, including the WHO analgesic ladder and numerous other drug and non-drug modalities (World Health Organization, 1990). The best choice of modality often changes as the patient's condition and the characteristics of the pain change. It is important that the effectiveness of analgesic modalities used separately or in combination be carefully assessed. The flowchart indicates the complexity of both the sources of pain and the types of modalities available for managing it. This guideline elaborates on the modalities, making recommendations about their appropriate use. **Whenever pain is present, clinicians should provide optimal pain relief by routinely assessing pain and treating it with one or more of the modalities described here.**

The WHO ladder (Figure 2) portrays a progression in the doses and types of analgesic drugs for effective pain management. When this

Figure 1. Flowchart: Continuing pain management in patients with cancer

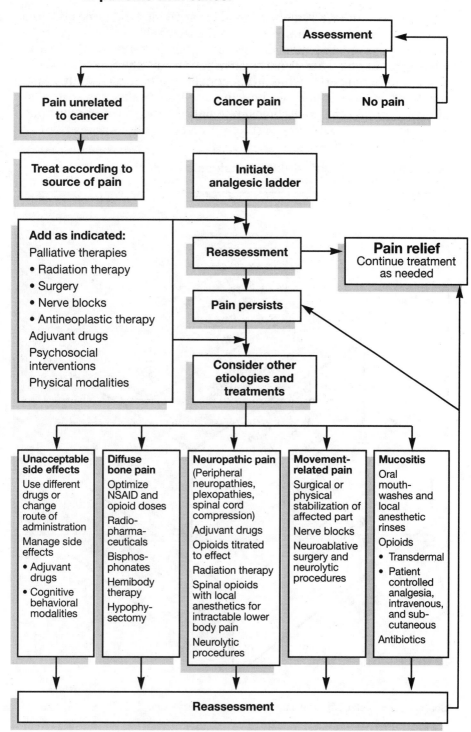

Assessment

Pain unrelated to cancer

Cancer pain

No pain

Treat according to source of pain

Initiate analgesic ladder

Add as indicated:
Palliative therapies
- Radiation therapy
- Surgery
- Nerve blocks
- Antineoplastic therapy

Adjuvant drugs

Psychosocial interventions

Physical modalities

Reassessment

Pain relief
Continue treatment as needed

Pain persists

Consider other etiologies and treatments

Unacceptable side effects

Use different drugs or change route of administration

Manage side effects
- Adjuvant drugs
- Cognitive behavioral modalities

Diffuse bone pain

Optimize NSAID and opioid doses

Radio-pharma-ceuticals

Bisphos-phonates

Hemibody therapy

Hypophy-sectomy

Neuropathic pain

(Peripheral neuropathies, plexopathies, spinal cord compression)

Adjuvant drugs

Opioids titrated to effect

Radiation therapy

Spinal opioids with local anesthetics for intractable lower body pain

Neurolytic procedures

Movement-related pain

Surgical or physical stabilization of affected part

Nerve blocks

Neuroablative surgery and neurolytic procedures

Mucositis

Oral mouth-washes and local anesthetic rinses

Opioids
- Transdermal
- Patient controlled analgesia, intravenous, and sub-cutaneous

Antibiotics

Reassessment

13

noninvasive approach is ineffective, alternative modalities include other routes of drug administration, nerve blocks, and ablative neurosurgery (Figure 3). As Figure 3 indicates, patients receiving treatments of varying degrees of invasiveness may also benefit from other modalities; the number of patients receiving these modalities either separately or in combination has not been well documented. The estimates presented in Figure 3 reflect various clinical populations and may not represent all settings and populations; furthermore, they do not necessarily

Figure 2. The WHO three-step analgesic ladder

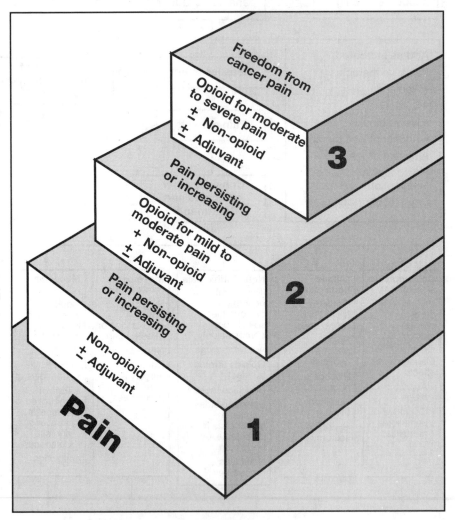

Source: World Health Organization, 1990. Used with permission.

Figure 3. Pain management strategies: a hierarchy

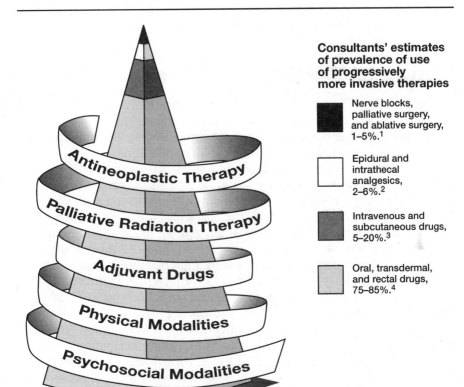

Consultants' estimates of prevalence of use of progressively more invasive therapies

Nerve blocks, palliative surgery, and ablative surgery, 1–5%.[1]

Epidural and intrathecal analgesics, 2–6%.[2]

Intravenous and subcutaneous drugs, 5–20%.[3]

Oral, transdermal, and rectal drugs, 75–85%.[4]

[1] Hiraga, Mizuguchi, and Takeda, 1991; Portenoy, 1993; Ventafridda, Caraceni, and Gamba, 1990.
[2] Hiraga, Mizuguchi, and Takeda, 1991; Ventafridda, Caraceni, and Gamba, 1990.
[3] Keller, 1984; Paice, 1993; Portenoy, 1993.
[4] Goisis, Gorini, Ratti, et al., 1989; Hiraga, Mizuguchi, and Takeda, 1991; Scug, Zech, and Dörr, 1990; Takeda, 1986; Ventafridda, Caraceni, and Gamba, 1990; Walker, Hoskin, Hanks, et al., 1988.

Note: The pyramid depicts a hierarchy of pain management strategies from least invasive (at the base) to most invasive (at the apex). Therapies depicted on the ribbon may benefit many patients who are receiving concurrent treatments at any level of invasiveness. Estimates presented in the sidebar are based on published data and consultants' estimates for various clinical populations in industrialized nations but may not reflect all settings and do not necessarily reflect what is optimal.

reflect what is optimal, but only a range of current opinions. There is a need for research to determine the effectiveness of many of these modalities used alone or in combination for different patient populations in various settings.

Barriers To Effective Pain Management

Pain management is often needlessly suboptimal (Table 2). Health care professionals are seldom trained in pain management, may not realize the importance of pain management or recognize that a patient is in pain, and may fear prescribing opioid medications.

Like some clinicians, patients and families may shun the use of opioids and, because of their fears of addiction and worries about tolerance, may not complain about pain or about poor pain relief. **Therefore, the panel recommends that clinicians include patient and family education about pain and its management in the treatment plan.**

Another barrier is that pain management has not traditionally been a priority of the health care system. Pain treatment may not be reimbursed or readily accessible, and institutions may be more concerned about a patient's possible opioid addiction or the diversion of controlled substances than about optimizing pain relief. Clinicians should reassure patients who are reluctant to report pain and who fear addiction and unmanageable side effects that there are many ways to relieve pain safely and effectively. Talking with clinicians knowledgeable about pain management and reading the consumer versions of this guideline (Jacox, Carr, Payne, et al., 1994, in press) should help patients and their families to overcome fears and concerns that hinder effective pain relief.

Problems related to the health care system and suggestions for resolving these are addressed extensively elsewhere (Angarola and Wray, 1989; Cain and Hammes, in press; Cleeland, Cleeland, Dar et al., 1986; Cleeland, 1987; Ferrell and Griffith, in press; Hammes and Cain, in press; Hill, 1993; Joranson, in press; Kolassa, in press; Shapiro, in press, a, b). Two of the problems—restrictive regulation of controlled substances and reimbursement policies—are discussed briefly here.

Legal Regulation of Opioids

The Federal government attempts to ensure the availability of opioid analgesics for legitimate medical and scientific purposes while controlling the abuse and illegal diversion of such substances (Shapiro, in press, a). The Controlled Substances Act (CSA) is one of the principal Federal laws that affects the use and availability of controlled substances, including opioid analgesics. The CSA provides for the registration of all handlers of controlled substances, as well as

Table 2. Barriers to cancer pain management

Problems related to health care professionals

Inadequate knowledge of pain management.[1]

Poor assessment of pain.[2]

Concern about regulation of controlled substances.[3]

Fear of patient addiction.[4]

Concern about side effects of analgesics.[5]

Concern about patients becoming tolerant to analgesics.[6]

Problems related to patients

Reluctance to report pain.[7]

Concern about distracting physicians from treatment of underlying disease.

Fear that pain means disease is worse.

Concern about not being a "good" patient.

Reluctance to take pain medications.[8]

Fear of addiction or of being thought of as an addict.

Worries about unmanageable side effects.

Concern about becoming tolerant to pain medications.

Problems related to the health care system

Low priority given to cancer pain treatment.[9]

Inadequate reimbursement.[10]

The most appropriate treatment may not be reimbursed or may be too costly for patients and families.

Restrictive regulation of controlled substances.[11]

Problems of availability of treatment or access to it.[12]

---

[1]Bonica, 1985; Cleeland, Cleeland, Dar, et al., 1986; Ferrell, Cronin Nash, and Warfield, 1992; Von Roenn, Cleeland, Gonin, et al., 1993.

[2]Grossman, Sheidler, Swedeen, et al., 1992; Von Roenn, Cleeland, Gonin, Hatfield, et al., 1993.

[3]Joranson, Cleeland, Weissman, et al., 1992; Shapiro, in press, a, b; Von Roenn, Cleeland, Gonin, et al., 1993; Weissman, Joranson, and Hopwood, 1991.

[4]Bonica, 1985; Ferrell, Cronin Nash, and Warfield, 1992; Marks and Sachar, 1973.

[5]Cleeland, Cleeland, Dar, et al., 1986; Von Roenn, Cleeland, Gonin, et al., 1993.

[6]Cleeland, Cleeland, Dar, et al., 1986; Shapiro, in press, a, b.

[7]Dar, Beach, Barden, et al., 1992; Levin, Cleeland, and Dar, 1985; Von Roenn, Cleeland, Gonin, et al., 1993; Ward, Goldberg, Miller-McCauley, et al., 1993.

[8]Cleeland, 1989; Dar, Beach, Barden, et al., 1992; Hodes, 1989; Joranson, in press; Levin, Cleeland, and Dar, 1985; Rimer, Levy, Keintz, et al., 1987; Von Roenn, Cleeland, Gonin, et al., 1993; Ward, Goldberg, Miller-McCauley, et al., 1993.

[9]Bonica, 1985; Max, 1990.

[10]Ferrell and Griffith, in press; Joranson, in press.

[11]Foley, 1985a; Joranson, Cleeland, Weissman, et al., 1992; Shapiro, in press, a, b; Weissman, Joranson, and Hopwood, 1991.

[12]Foley, 1985a.

for the labeling, order forms, recordkeeping, and reporting of substances or their use. These activities enable enforcement agencies to identify manufacturers, distributors, clinicians, and pharmacists who divert controlled substances for illicit uses. The CSA also includes provisions that explicitly aim to avoid interference with the availability of U.S. Food and Drug Administration (FDA)-approved drugs for legitimate purposes. The CSA does not restrict a clinician's medical decision about which drug to prescribe, in what amounts, or for what duration, although it does prohibit physicians from prescribing opioids to maintain narcotic addiction unless the physician is separately registered to treat addiction. "Addict" is defined in the CSA as one who habitually uses an opioid drug so as to endanger public health or safety or one who has lost control over opioid use (Controlled Substances Act, 21 U.S.C., sec. 802). This definition rarely applies to a patient being treated with opioids for cancer pain (Kanner and Foley, 1981). Furthermore, Federal controlled substances regulations clarify that the Federal law is not intended to impose limitations on a physician's ability to prescribe opioid analgesics to persons with intractable pain in situations where no relief or cure is possible or none has been found after reasonable efforts (21 CFR 1306.07(c)).

State laws vary greatly, and many restrict or regulate the prescribing of opioids in the treatment of pain in ways that Federal law does not. For example, many State drug diversion laws contain ill-defined terms that in effect restrict opioid prescribing (Joranson, 1990). Other State laws also regulate pain treatment by restricting medication prescriptions to a specific number of dosage units or to a 1-month supply, or by monitoring the prescription of controlled substances through multiple-copy prescription programs. WHO has observed that although multiple-copy prescription programs are intended to reduce careless prescribing, "Health care workers may be reluctant to prescribe, stock or dispense opioids as they feel that there is a possibility of their professional licenses being suspended or revoked by the governing authority in cases where large quantities of opioids are provided to an individual, even though the medical need for such drugs can be proved" (World Health Organization, 1990). In States with formal cancer pain initiatives, health professionals have worked with State agencies to identify and remove legal impediments to the use of controlled substances for cancer pain (Dahl, Joranson, Engber, et al., 1988).

A 1990 revision of the Uniform Controlled Substances Act addresses the legitimate use of controlled substances by recognizing that the prescribing, administering, and dispensing of opioid analgesics for intractable pain is part of professional medical treatment. It states that if terms such as *addict, habitual user, and drug-dependent person* are used in States' statutes, definitions of these terms should clearly indicate that they do not apply to patients receiving controlled substances pursuant to a practitioner's order (Uniform Controlled Substances Act, 1990). Each State legislature has received the revision from the Uniform Law Commissioners.

The panel recommends that laws and regulatory policies aimed at diversion control not hamper the appropriate use of opioid analgesics for cancer pain. Clinicians are responsible for knowing how controlled substances are regulated in their States. Such information can be obtained from State medical, nursing, and pharmacy licensing boards (see Angarola, 1990; Joranson, 1990; Shapiro, in press, a, for additional information on the regulation of analgesic drugs).

Cost and Reimbursement for Pain Management_____

Determining the overall cost of pain management is difficult because it generally is not separated from other treatment costs, but rather is included as part of the patient's stay in the hospital or an outpatient visit. Components of pain management costs and a comparison of analgesic drug costs are discussed by Ferrell and Griffith (in press) and Kolassa (in press).

Access to professional services, prescription drugs, and medical equipment is usually necessary for effective pain care (Joranson, in press). Reimbursement or lack of it influences the way in which pain is treated, where it is treated, and the supportive care that is available (Yasco and Verfurth, 1992). Reimbursement policies of third-party payers for pain management differ substantially, and many people with cancer are uninsured or underinsured. According to one report (American Cancer Society, 1989), low-income people experience greater pain and suffering from cancer than do other Americans, and a disproportionate share of people with little or no insurance are minorities. For those who are insured, reimbursement policies may favor the use of more expensive pain management modalities over less expensive ones. Medicare, for example, does not reimburse for outpatient oral analgesics but will reimburse for pain management in an inpatient facility. Thus, "a person may well have reimbursement for the $4,000.00 cost of patient controlled analgesia (PCA) morphine but will have no coverage for $100.00 of oral morphine solution" (Ferrell and Griffith, in press). Joranson (in press) has reported on the variation in the policies of private payers and health maintenance organizations, in which policies are often unclear about or offer minimal coverage for pain management. Reimbursement policies on pain management should be studied to enable further understanding of those that promote the most cost effective pain management.

Clinicians should consider a patient's ability to pay for treatment. The costs of medication and other treatments may overburden a patient with limited financial resources and result in compromises between adherence to the prescribed regimen and other financial responsibilities (Brand, Smith, and Grand, 1977). Costs of analgesic drugs, for example, including many that are equally effective for pain management, vary dramatically (Kolassa, in press). For example, an analysis of the costs of NSAIDs included in the drug tables of this guideline showed that the retail price of NSAIDs (excluding acetaminophen and aspirin) in 1992 ranged from $10.50 to $127.80 for a 30-day supply (Kolassa, in press). Although the primary concern of the clinician is to manage pain effectively, the ability to do this may be influenced by the patient's economic status. **Therefore, clinicians should collaborate with patients and families, taking cost of drugs and technologies into account when selecting pain management strategies.**

Methods Used To Develop the Guideline

This guideline was developed by an interdisciplinary, expert panel, commissioned by AHCPR, that comprises practitioners in nursing, medicine, pharmacy, psychology, and physical therapy; health care consumers; and an ethicist.

The panel used four processes to develop the guidelines. First, it undertook an extensive and interdisciplinary clinical review of current needs, therapeutic practices and principles, and emerging technologies for cancer pain control. This process included a review of all pertinent guidelines and standards, the solicitation of information and opinions from external consultants, and an open forum (announced in the *Federal Register* and held in Washington, DC, on September 5, 1991) to receive the broadest possible input from concerned parties.

Second, the panel performed a comprehensive scientific review of the field to define the existing knowledge base and evaluate critically the assumptions and common wisdom in the field. Although the primary focus of the review was on cancer pain, the panel also reviewed the pain literature on HIV positive/AIDS. When there were few studies available that tested the use of interventions with various populations of cancer patients, studies conducted on other clinical populations were used as supplementary scientific evidence. The panel examined studies on patients of all ages. It performed a best-evidence synthesis of the scientific evidence, including a meta-analysis when sufficient numbers of experimental studies were found in the literature. Nineteen data bases were searched, and approximately 9,600 citations were screened. Six hundred twenty-five research studies were critiqued for scientific merit, and 550 were included in tables of evidence for the various interventions.

Attachment A gives ratings of strength of the scientific evidence for interventions, along with the types and ratings for evidence of the specific interventions included in the guidelines. Briefly, the *strength and consistency of evidence* for recommendations describes the evidence and notes whether it is generally consistent or inconsistent. Strength of evidence ranges from A (strongest) to D (little or no systematic empirical evidence).

When the strength of evidence is A or B, the panel's recommendations are based primarily on the evidence. When the strength of recommendation is C or D, the panel used the available empirical evidence but based their recommendations primarily on expert judgment. When the recommendation is a statement of panel opinion regarding desirable practice and there is evidence that the practice is not commonly being followed, the term "panel consensus" is used.

Third, guideline drafts were developed by members of the panel, consultants, and panel staff. In all, 17 drafts were written.

Fourth, the panel initiated peer review of two drafts of the guideline and field tested a draft with intended users in clinical sites. Comments were reviewed and incorporated into the final guideline. The patient brochure was developed by panel members and field tested with 69 patients and six clinicians.

Four hundred sixty-eight consultants, peer reviewers, and site testers reviewed and contributed to the development of the guideline. The entire process was anchored by the panel, which met six times over a period of 2 years.

Organization of Guideline

Users of this guideline can easily refer to sections of immediate interest. It begins with a discussion of pain assessment and then presents methods of pain control. These methods appear in separate sections dealing with the pharmacologic management of pain, the use of psychosocial and physical modalities, and the use of anesthetic and surgical interventions and radiation therapy. One chapter discusses procedure-related pain in adults and children. Another addresses pain in special populations, including infants and children, the elderly, known or suspected substance abusers, minorities, HIV positive/AIDS patients, and people with psychiatric problems. The final section discusses institutional responsibility for effective pain management. Attachment A contains tables of scientific evidence for the interventions. Attachment B contains pain assessment instruments for adults and children. Attachment C includes sample relaxation exercises. A glossary, as well as lists of consultants, peer reviewers, and site testers of the guideline are also provided. To derive maximal benefit, clinicians should read the entire guideline.

2 Assessment of Pain in the Patient With Cancer

Recommendations

7. Health professionals should ask about pain, and the patient's self-report should be the primary source of assessment. (B)

8. Clinicians should assess pain with easily administered rating scales and should document the efficacy of pain relief at regular intervals after starting or changing treatment. Documentation forms should be readily accessible to all clinicians involved in the patient's care. (Panel Consensus)

9. Clinicians should teach patients and their families to use assessment tools in their homes in order to promote continuity of effective pain management across all settings. (Panel Consensus)

10. The initial evaluation of pain should include:

   ■ A detailed history, including an assessment of pain intensity and characteristics.

   ■ A physical examination.

   ■ A psychosocial assessment.

   ■ A diagnostic evaluation of signs and symptoms associated with the common cancer pain syndromes. (Panel Consensus)

11. Clinicians should be aware of common pain syndromes: this prompt recognition may hasten therapy and minimize the morbidity of unrelieved pain. (B)

12. Changes in pain patterns or the development of new pain should trigger a diagnostic evaluation and modification of the treatment plan. (Panel Consensus)

Assessment of pain in the cancer patient is imperative for all health care professionals because failure to assess pain can lead to its undertreatment. The critical role of the assessment of cancer pain was highlighted in a 1993 study of 897 oncologists who, collectively in the previous 6 months, had managed more than 70,000 cancer patients. According to these physicians, poor pain assessment was the greatest barrier to effective cancer pain management in their own practices (Von Roenn, Cleeland, Gonin, et al., 1993). Because of the multiple possible causes of pain, careful evaluation of pain is required.

Initial Pain Assessment

The initial assessment should occur with each new report of pain and should focus on identifying the cause of the pain and developing a pain management plan. Subsequent assessments should evaluate the effectiveness of the plan and, if pain is unrelieved, determine whether the cause is related to the progression of disease, a new cause of pain, or the cancer treatment.

The initial evaluation of pain should include:

■ **Detailed history, including an assessment of the pain intensity and character.**

■ **Physical examination, emphasizing the neurologic examination.**

■ **Psychosocial assessment.**

■ **Appropriate diagnostic workup to determine the cause of the pain.**

Attention to detail is important: a delayed or incorrect diagnosis, particularly with a syndrome such as spinal cord compression, can result in increased morbidity, needless pain and suffering, or both. The initial assessment should provide a detailed description of each type of pain (Table 3).

Health professionals should ask about pain, and the patient's self-report should be the primary source of assessment. The self-report should include a description of the pain; its location, intensity/severity, and aggravating and relieving factors; and the patient's cognitive response to pain. Neither behavior nor vital signs should be used in lieu of a self-report (Beyer, McGrath, and Berde, 1990). **It is best to use brief, easy-to-use assessment tools that reliably document pain intensity and pain relief and to relate these to other dimensions of pain such as mood.** (Examples of both brief and comprehensive pain inventories are included in Attachment B.) One routine clinical approach to pain assessment and management is summarized by the mnemonic "ABCDE":

A Ask about pain regularly.

Assess pain systematically.

B Believe the patient and family in their reports of pain and what relieves it.

C Choose pain control options appropriate for the patient, family, and setting.

D Deliver interventions in a timely, logical, and coordinated fashion.

E Empower patients and their families.

Enable them to control their course to the greatest extent possible.

Table 3. Initial pain assessment

A. Assessment of pain intensity and character

1. **Onset and temporal pattern**—When did your pain start? How often does it occur? Has its intensity changed?
2. **Location**—Where is your pain? Is there more than one site?
3. **Description**—What does your pain feel like? What words would you use to describe your pain?
4. **Intensity**—On a scale of 0 to 10, with 0 being no pain and 10 being the worst pain you can imagine, how much does it hurt right now? How much does it hurt at its worst? How much does it hurt at its best?
5. **Aggravating and relieving factors**—What makes your pain better? What makes your pain worse?
6. **Previous treatment**—What types of treatments have you tried to relieve your pain? Were they and are they effective?
7. **Effect**—How does the pain affect physical and social function?

B. Psychosocial assessment
Psychosocial assessment should include the following:

1. Effect and understanding of the cancer diagnosis and cancer treatment on the patient and the caregiver.
2. The meaning of the pain to the patient and the family.
3. Significant past instances of pain and their effect on the patient.
4. The patient's typical coping responses to stress or pain.
5. The patient's knowledge of, curiosity about, preferences for, and expectations about pain management methods.
6. The patient's concerns about using controlled substances such as opioids, anxiolytics, or stimulants.
7. The economic effect of the pain and its treatment.
8. Changes in mood that have occurred as a result of the pain (e.g., depression, anxiety).

C. Physical and neurologic examination

1. Examine site of pain and evaluate common referral patterns.
2. Perform pertinent neurologic evaluation.
   - Head and neck pain—cranial nerve and fundoscopic evaluation.
   - Back and neck pain—motor and sensory function in limbs; rectal and urinary sphincter function.

D. Diagnostic evaluation

1. Evaluate recurrence or progression of disease or tissue injury related to cancer treatment.
   - Tumor markers and other blood tests.
   - Radiologic studies.
   - Neurophysiologic (e.g., electromyography) testing.
2. Perform appropriate radiologic studies and correlate normal and abnormal findings with physical and neurologic examination.
3. Recognize limitations of diagnostic studies.
   - Bone scan—false negatives in myeloma, lymphoma, previous radiotherapy sites.
   - CT scan—good definition of bone and soft tissue but difficult to image entire spine.
   - MRI scan—bone definition not as good as CT; better images of spine and brain.

In the initial assessment, document the onset and temporal pattern of the pain. Ask patients to point to the exact location of the pain on themselves or the clinician (The Brief Pain Inventory and the Initial Pain Assessment Tool in Attachment B). Determine whether the pain radiates or spreads to other parts of the body.

Ask patients to describe their pain: the descriptive words they use can provide valuable clues as to the cause. For example, patients who describe back pain that radiates like a tight band around their chest and worsens with coughing or defecation should be evaluated for potential spinal cord compression, a complication of vertebral body metastasis. Patients who describe their pain as "burning" or "tingling" are likely to have a neuropathic cause of pain—particularly when it is associated with subjective numbness, loss of sensation, and weakness (Elliott and Foley, 1989).

Three commonly used self-report assessment tools (Figure 4) are:

- Simple Descriptive Pain Intensity Scale.

- 0-10 Numeric Pain Intensity Scale.

- Visual Analog Scale (VAS).

Figure 4. Pain intensity scales

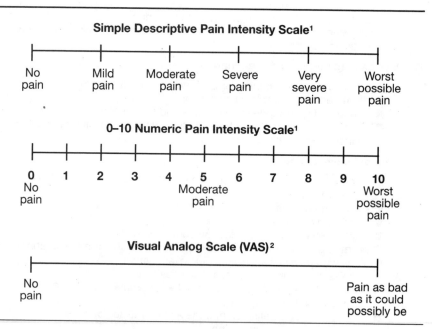

[1] If used as a graphic rating scale, a 10 cm baseline is recommended.
[2] A 10-cm baseline is recommended for VAS scales.

Source: Acute Pain Management Guideline Panel, 1992.

If the patient understands the scale and is capable of answering and if end points and adjective descriptors are carefully selected, each of these instruments can be valid and reliable (Gracely and Wolskee, 1983; Houde, 1982; Sriwatanakul, Kelvie, and Lasagna, 1982).

An assessment of pain intensity should include an evaluation of not only the present pain intensity but also pain at its least and worst. Knowing factors that aggravate or relieve pain helps clinicians to design a pain treatment plan. The initial pain assessment should elicit information about changes in activities of daily living, including work and recreational activities, sleep patterns, mobility, appetite, sexual functioning, and mood.

A psychosocial assessment should emphasize the effect of pain on patients and their families, as well as patients' preferences among pain management methods. Patients who are able to answer should be asked about the effectiveness of past and present pain treatments, such as antineoplastic therapy or specific pharmacologic and nonpharmacologic therapies.

The clinician should perform a physical and neurologic examination related to the pain report (see below, Assessment of Common Cancer Pain Syndromes). The painful area should be carefully examined to determine if palpation or manipulation of the site exacerbates the pain. Common sites of pain referral should be evaluated (e.g., shoulder pain may emanate from subdiaphragmatic abdominal sources; knee and hip pain may be referred from lumbar spine lesions). In addition, the patient should be observed for cues that indicate pain, e.g., distorted posture, impaired mobility, guarding the painful area, restricted movement of a limb, anxiety, attention seeking, or depression. However, absence of these behaviors should not be interpreted to mean that the patient has no pain.

Neurologic examination should be focused. For example, pain in the head and neck region requires careful cranial nerve examination to exclude intracranial pathology and lesions at the base of the skull, that may require definition by specialized magnetic resonance imaging (MRI) or computed tomography (CT). Neck or back pain require careful motor, sensory, and reflex examination of the arms and legs, as well as evaluation of rectal and urinary sphincter function to exclude plexopathy and spinal cord lesions.

Appropriate diagnostic tests should be performed to determine the cause of the pain and the extent of disease, and patients should be offered analgesia to facilitate these evaluations (e.g., to allow the patient to lie flat for CT or MRI scans). It is important to correlate the results of these studies with physical and neurologic findings to assure that appropriate areas of the body have been imaged and that identified abnormalities do in fact explain the patient's pain. Pain may be the first sign of tumor recurrence or progression and may appear or increase before changes are evident in imaging studies; therefore, imaging studies may have to be repeated.

Ongoing Pain Assessment

The assessment of the patient's pain and the efficacy of the treatment plan should be ongoing, and the pain reports should be documented. Simply to record a patient's responses to the question "How is your pain?" invites misunderstanding and hinders quantification.

Pain should be assessed and documented:

- **At regular intervals after starting the treatment plan.**

- **With each new report of pain.**

- **At a suitable interval after each pharmacologic or nonpharmacologic intervention, such as 15 to 30 minutes after parenteral drug therapy and 1 hour after oral administration.**

Occasionally, discrepancies between behaviors and a patient's self-report of pain may occur. For example, patients may describe pain as an 8, on a scale of 0 to 10, while smiling and walking freely, or conversely, as a 2 while experiencing tachycardia, splinting, and sweating, although this is less usual. These discrepancies may result from several factors, including the effectiveness of the patient's coping skills (see Chapter 4). The patient who uses distraction and relaxation techniques may engage in diversionary activities while still experiencing severe pain; in fact, this is a goal of many behavioral pain therapies. Patients may deny severe pain for a variety of reasons, including a perception that stoicism is expected or rewarded or a fear that the pain symbolizes disease progression. Similarly, patients managed with as-needed analgesia may perceive that medication will be given only if the pain score is very high. When discussing pain assessment and control with patients, members of the health care team should emphasize the importance of a factual report, thereby avoiding both stoicism and exaggeration. If anxiety or other concerns are significant, patients should be asked to rate their emotional distress separately from their pain, using similar scales (see Pain Distress Scales in Attachment B). They also may be asked to rate their mood or the effectiveness of analgesic therapies (see the Memorial Pain Assessment Card in Attachment B). When discrepancies between behaviors and self-reports of pain occur, these differences should be discussed with the patient, and the pain management plan should then be revised.

Most cancer patients are treated for pain in outpatient and home care settings. Plans should be made to ensure ongoing assessment of the pain and the effectiveness of treatments in these settings. Patients can keep a log of their pain intensity scores and report these scores during followup visits or through telephone followup. **In addition, patients should be taught to report changes in their pain or any new pain so that appropriate reassessment and changes in the treatment plan can be initiated.**

Patients unable to communicate effectively with staff require special consideration (see Chapter 7). Even patients previously able to communicate may be unable to do so as their disease progresses. Aggressive efforts should be made to find a translator for the non-English-speaking patient to determine a convenient way to assess pain. Many of the pain assessment tools have already been translated (Beyer and Wells, 1993; Cleeland and Syrjala, 1992).

When developing a treatment plan, members of the health care team should pay particular attention to the preferences and needs of patients whose education or cultural traditions may impede effective communication (see Chapter 7 for additional discussion). Certain cultures have strong beliefs about pain and its management, and members of these cultures may hesitate to report unrelieved pain or may have specific preferences for pain-relieving measures. When developing a treatment plan, clinicians should be aware of the unique needs and circumstances of patients from different age groups or various ethnic and cultural backgrounds.

Assessment of Common Cancer Pain Syndromes

Patients can experience acute or chronic pain from their cancer, diagnostic procedures, treatment, or preexisting conditions. Thus, patients should be carefully assessed to ensure that the cause of pain is established whenever possible and treated appropriately.

Some causes of cancer pain are relatively easy to diagnose and treat (e.g., pathologic fractures). **However, clinicians treating patients with cancer should also be able to recognize readily the common pain syndromes that may cause intractable pain and that may signal disease recurrence in order to optimize therapy and minimize the morbidity of unrelieved pain.** Furthermore, because many intractable pain problems involve neurologic structures (e.g., epidural spinal cord compression; metastatic brachial and lumbosacral plexopathy), prompt recognition and treatment of these syndromes may also minimize neurologic impairment (Elliott and Foley, 1989).

Bone Metastases_____

Multiple myeloma and cancers of the breast, prostate, and lung account for a large majority of bone metastases. The most common sites of bone metastasis include the vertebrae, pelvis, femur, and skull. Distal extremity metastases are uncommon (Malawer and Delaney, 1989). The most frequent symptom is pain, although 25 percent of patients with bone metastases have no symptoms (Wagner, 1984). Pain may result from direct tumor involvement of bone with activation of local nociceptors, or compression of adjacent nerves, vascular structures, and soft tissue. Because patients often have multiple sites of bone metastases, multiple areas of pain are common. Pain is usually described as dull and aching, is usually localized to the area of metastasis, and is increased by movement. However, spine metastases may impinge upon nerve roots and result in radicular pain. Patients with metastases to the base of the skull may complain of headache; pain on head movement; and face, neck, or shoulder pain (Greenberg, Deck, Vikram, et al., 1981). Besides pain and immobility, complications of bone metastases include fractures, hypercalcemia, and spinal cord compression. Pathologic fractures occur most commonly in cancers of the breast, lung, kidney, and thyroid and in multiple myeloma, usually in the proximal femur or humerus (Oda and Schurman, 1983). Hypercalcemia is most often observed in cancers of the breast, lung, and kidney and in multiple myeloma.

The diagnosis of bone metastasis is established by radiographic confirmation and, rarely, biopsy. Radionuclide scintigraphy and magnetic resonance imaging are the most sensitive means of detecting bone metastases, often demonstrating abnormalities before those seen on plain radiographs. Plain radiographs showing typical lytic, blastic, or mixed lesions are usually diagnostic and easily distinguished from lesions resulting from nonmetastatic causes (Wilner, 1982). However, plain radiographs and bone scintigraphy may be negative early in the course of myeloma, in some osseous metastases, and at sites of previously radiated bone (Kelly and Payne, 1991). Magnetic resonance imaging may be helpful in such cases when bone involvement is suspected.

Epidural Metastases/Spinal Cord Compression_____

Epidural metastasis is the most ominous complication of bone metastasis to the vertebral spine and is a medical emergency. Failure to diagnose and treat this condition will lead to permanent neurologic deficits due to spinal cord dysfunction. Early diagnosis, before overt neurologic deficits, should result in improved outcome (Byrne, 1992). Epidural metastasis is a common complication in patients with breast, prostate, or lung cancer; multiple myeloma; renal cell carcinoma; or melanoma. The tumor enters the epidural space by contiguous spread from adjacent vertebral metastases in the vast majority of cases (Rodriguez and Dinapoli, 1980). The remaining cases arise from the direct invasion of retroperitoneal tumor or tumor located in the posterior thorax through adjacent intervertebral foramina or, rarely, from bloodborne seeding of the epidural space. The pain is usually midline, but patients whose tumor involves nerve roots have sharp or shooting pain in a radicular distribution. Untreated, the pain slowly intensifies with a mean duration of 7 weeks from the onset of pain to the onset of neurologic deficits due to spinal cord compression (Gilbert, Kim, and Posner, 1978). Signs of spinal cord compression include motor, sensory, and autonomic (e.g., bladder and bowel) dysfunction.

More than 70 percent of patients with spinal cord compression have an abnormal plain radiograph in the region of pain (compression fracture, blastic, or lytic metastases) (Portenoy, Lipton, and Foley, 1987). Because pain is such a reliable early sign, epidural metastases can often be diagnosed and treated before neurologic deficits develop. Patients with persistent back pain in the region of abnormality on plain spine radiograph, with or without neurologic deficits, should undergo evaluation with MRI. Patients with progressive back or neck pain whose plain radiograph is normal should also undergo an imaging study of the epidural space, even if their neurologic examination is normal. Administration of analgesics and corticosteroids constitutes the mainstay of pharmacologic therapy. Radiation therapy or surgical excision followed by radiation therapy are the two standard treatments.

Metastases to the Skull

Table 4 lists common metastases to the skull, which often cause pain in patients with cancer.

Plexopathies

Cervical, brachial, and lumbosacral plexi can be sources of intractable pain in cancer patients (Elliott and Foley, 1989). Pain is produced when these structures are infiltrated by tumor or compressed by fibrosis after radiation therapy to adjacent structures. Pain tends to be less prominent in radiation-induced plexopathies than in tumor-related ones. Traction injury related to the positioning of a patient during a prolonged operation may also produce brachial plexopathy.

Pain originating in the cervical plexus often occurs as an aching discomfort that may radiate into the neck and occiput. It is most commonly caused by metastases to the cervical lymph nodes or the local extension of primary head and neck tumors.

Table 4. Metastases to the skull

Type of metastases	Signs and symptoms
Middle fossa syndrome	Similar to trigeminal neuralgia, i.e., numbness, paresthesia, and pain referred to the second or third divisions of the fifth nerve, except that objective signs of neuropathy, e.g., corresponding sensory deficits and masseter weakness, may be present. Diplopia, dysarthria, headache, and dysphagia may develop as well.
Jugular foramen syndrome	Occipital pain often radiating to the vertex and ipsilateral shoulder or neck; may be accompanied by local tenderness and exacerbation with movement of the head. Neurologic signs consistent with dysfunction of cranial nerves IX through XII and Horner's syndrome may be present. Lancinating throat pain (glossopharyngeal neuralgia) has been observed in association with the above symptoms or as the sole complaint.
Clivus metastases	Vertex headache exacerbated by neck flexion; may be accompanied by either unilateral or bilateral cranial nerve dysfunction (IV through XXII).
Orbital metastases	Retro-orbital or frontal headache often with diplopia, visual loss, proptosis, and extraocular nerve palsies.
Parasellar metastases	Symptoms similar to those of orbital metastases.
Sphenoid sinus metastases	Bifrontal headache radiating to both temples with intermittent retro-orbital pain. Nasal stuffiness, diplopia, and a unilateral or bilateral VI cranial nerve palsy may be present.
Occipital condyle invasion	Severe occipital pain that is exacerbated by movement and that may be accompanied by XII cranial nerve dysfunction.
Odontoid fractures	Usually caused by tumor or metastasis to atlas bone. Risk of spinal cord compression due to vertebral instability.

Source: Adapted from Elliot and Foley, 1989; Greenberg, Deck, Vikram, et al., 1981.

Brachial plexopathy is a common complication of breast and lung cancer and lymphoma, but it can also be caused by metastasis to the brachial plexus from a remote primary tumor (Kori, Foley, and Posner, 1981). Pain occurs in up to 85 percent of patients with brachial plexus involvement and may precede weakness or sensory loss by months (Foley, 1987). When the upper plexus is damaged by tumor, pain usually begins in the shoulder and is associated with shooting or electrical sensations in the thumb and index finger. When the lower plexus is involved, as is more common, pain begins in the shoulder and radiates into the elbow, arm, and medial forearm, and into the fourth and fifth digits. In about 25 percent of patients, both upper and lower divisions are involved. Compared with tumor-related plexopathy, radiation damage to the brachial plexus causes less severe pain, distributed initially in the upper division.

Epidural extension may occur in up to 50 percent of patients with superior pulmonary sulcus ("Pancoast") tumors (Kanner and Foley, 1981). Epidural disease is more likely to occur when the entire plexus is involved and Horner's syndrome is present, which indicates medial and paraspinal spread of tumor. Lymphoma may produce brachial plexopathy and spinal cord compression in the absence of vertebral body erosion. CT and MRI of the brachial plexus and epidural spaces are the diagnostic procedures of choice, and are essential to define the extent of disease and to determine the appropriate radiation ports.

The lumbosacral plexus, embedded in the psoas muscle, may be invaded by tumors of the abdomen and pelvis. Colorectal, endometrial, and renal cancers, as well as sarcomas and lymphomas, may invade this plexus by direct spread. However, 25 percent of lumbosacral plexopathies are metastatic (Jaeckle, Young, and Foley, 1985). Pain is usually felt in the lower abdomen, buttock, and leg. Infiltration of the sacral plexus may produce perineal and perirectal pain, which is exacerbated by sitting and lying prone. Pain typically precedes, by weeks or even months, the neurologic signs of weakness, sensory loss, or urinary incontinence. Abdominal and pelvic CT or MRI may provide the diagnosis and allow definition of radiation portals. Similar to patients with brachial plexopathy, patients with diffuse or bilateral lumbosacral plexus involvement may have an epidural extension of tumor, in which case, MRI of the epidural space is also required. Epidural disease of the cauda equina or leptomeningeal tumor may produce a clinical syndrome similar to lumbosacral plexopathy (Elliott and Foley, 1989).

Pain may precede overt neurologic signs in spinal cord compression, plexopathies, and spinal metastasis. Prompt recognition of these syndromes and institution of appropriate treatment can avoid paralysis and incontinence.

Peripheral Neuropathies

Peripheral nerves can be compressed or infiltrated by tumor or constricted by fibrosis, which in rare instances is a complication of radiation treatment. They may also be damaged by neurotoxic chemotherapy or by cutaneous incisions and the retraction of tissues during surgery (Table 5).

Myeloma may cause a progressive painful neuropathy in about 15 percent of patients. In as many as 8 of 10 such patients, neuropathy precedes the onset of other symptoms (Davis and Drachman, 1972). This sensorimotor neuropathy is characterized by distal paraesthesias,

33

Table 5. Common cancer pain syndromes due to peripheral nerve injury

Pain syndrome	Associated signs and symptoms	Affected nerves
Tumor infiltration of a peripheral nerve	Constant, burning pain with dysesthesia in an area of sensory loss Pain is radicular and often unilateral	Peripheral
Postradical neck dissection	Tight, burning sensation in the area of sensory loss Dysesthesias and shocklike pain may be present Second type of pain may occur mimicking a drooped shoulder syndrome	Cervical plexus
Postmastectomy pain	Tight, constricting, burning pain in the posterior arm, axilla, and anterior chest wall Pain exacerbated by arm movement	Intercostobrachial
Postthoracotomy pain	Aching sensation in the distribution of the incision with sensory loss with or without autonomic changes Often exquisite point tenderness at the most medial and apical points of the scar with a specific trigger point Secondary reflex sympathetic dystrophy may develop	Intercostal
Postnephrectomy pain	Numbness, fullness, or heaviness in the flank, anterior abdomen, and groin Dysesthesias are common	Superficial flank
Postlimb amputation	Phantom limb pain usually occurs after pain in the same site before amputation Stump pain occurs at the site of the surgical scar, several months to years after surgery. It is characterized by a burning dysesthetic sensation that is exacerbated by movement	Peripheral endings and their central projections

sensory loss, weakness, and muscle wasting, and it may occasionally ascend upward in a manner similar to Guillain-Barré syndrome.

Vincristine, cisplatin, and taxol produce dose-related peripheral neuropathies, usually manifested as dysesthesia in the feet and later (as the neuropathy progresses) in the hands; continuous burning pain is rarely a problem. Vincristine neuropathy may also give rise to cranial neuralgias, including jaw claudication. Treatment of chemotherapy-related neuropathy involves decreasing or stopping the offending agent (when possible) and the use of analgesics.

Pain syndrome	Associated signs and symptoms	Affected nerves
Chemotherapy-induced peripheral neuropathy	Painful paresthesias and dysesthesias Hyporeflexia Less frequently: motor and sensory loss; rarely: autonomic dysfunction Commonly associated with the vinca alkaloids, cisplatin, and Taxol	Distal areas of peripheral (e.g., polyneuropathy)
Radiation-induced peripheral nerve tumors	May promote malignant fibrosarcoma Painful, enlarging mass in a previously irradiated area Patients with neurofibromatosis more susceptible	Superficial and deep
Cranial neuropathies	Severe head pain with cranial nerve dysfunction Leptomeningeal disease Base of skull metastasis	Cranial V, VII, IX, X, XI, XII are most common
Acute and postherpetic neuropathy	Painful paresthesia and dysesthesia Constant burning and aching pain Shocklike paroxysmal pain Immunosuppression from disease or treatment is a risk factor; postherpetic neuropathy incidence increases with age	Thoracic and cranial (VI) are most common

Note: See Chapters 3, 4, and 5 for treatment of cancer-related neuropathies.

Source: Adapted from Foley, 1985b; Kanner, 1985; Payne 1985.

In the absence of recurrent tumor, persistent pain following surgery may result from intraoperative injury to cutaneous or deeper nerves. Postsurgical pain syndromes are characterized by either persistent pain after the surgical procedure or recurrent pain after the initial surgical pain has resolved. The clinical characteristics relate to the location and extent of nerve injury (Kelly and Payne, 1991). Treatment of these syndromes involves the use of analgesics and, occasionally, regional nerve blocks.

Table 6. Common causes of abdominal pain

Obstruction of small or large bowel.

Occlusion of blood flow to visceral organs (e.g., liver, kidney, large and small bowel).

Thrombosis and engorgement of splenic or renal veins.

Omental metastasis.

Volvulus of the small intestine.

Infectious or chemical peritonitis.

Metastasis or lymphomatous liver distention.

Acute and Postherpetic Neuralgia

Varicella-zoster virus infection or reactivation ("shingles") is more likely to occur in patients with cancer than in the general population because of the higher incidence of immunosuppression in the former. Zoster neuralgia may cause acute and chronic pain (Rusthoven, Ahlgren, Elhakim, et al., 1988). Disseminated zoster is twice as likely to occur in patients with progressive tumor than those in remission (Rusthoven, Ahlgren, Elhakim, et al., 1988). Thoracic and cranial dermatomes are most commonly affected, and the incidence of postherpetic neuralgia (pain after healing of rash) increases with age (Watson, Evans, Reed, et al., 1982).

Varicella-zoster virus infection is characterized by a burning, aching pain. Lancinating or shocklike pain may be superimposed in the area of the crusted (or healed) herpetic skin lesions, in which there is usually sensory loss. Hyperpathia may be profound. For acute zoster, antiviral therapies in combination with analgesics are recommended. For postherpetic neuralgia, antiviral therapies are of limited use, and therapies for neuropathic pain are used (see Chapter 3). Empiric observations suggest that nerve blocks during acute herpes zoster infection reduce pain, shorten the acute episode, and prevent the emergence of postherpetic neuralgia (Bonica, 1990). Treatment approaches for neuropathic pain are discussed later (see also Figure 1).

Abdominal Pain

Abdominal tumors are frequently characterized by pain that is colicky, worse after eating, and associated with nausea. Pain may be referred widely throughout the abdomen to distant cutaneous sites (e.g., shoulder, neck, and back). Patients with tumors of the small or large intestine occasionally have a combination of obstruction, pain,

Table 7. Assessment of mucositis

Examine lips and all mucosal surfaces for number, size, and location of lesions. Pain intensity is usually related to the degree of tissue damage.

Include assessment of local edema and erythema as well as preexisting periodontal disease that may also be painful.

Ask patient to identify painful or burning areas; even if there is no apparent tissue damage, these may become involved later.

Culture suspicious lesions to rule out concomitant infection (bacterial, viral, fungal) that may intensify pain and delay healing.

Evaluate patient's ability to swallow (including oral analgesics), and restrict oral intake if necessary.

Repeat the assessment frequently because clinical signs and symptoms may change.

and hematemesis or rectal bleeding. Common causes of abdominal pain for these patients are listed in Table 6.

Patients with cancer are vulnerable to developing the same nonmalignant medical and surgical causes of abdominal pain, such as appendicitis, cholecystitis, and pancreatitis, as are individuals without cancer. Opioid analgesic therapy is often constrained in this group of patients by nausea, constipation, and ileus related to tumor-related bowel obstruction. Treatment of abdominal pain with nerve blocks is discussed in Chapter 5.

Mucositis

Mucositis can occur in any patient receiving cytotoxic chemotherapy or radiation to the head and neck. In patients receiving chemotherapy, the incidence and severity of mucosal toxicity is influenced by the individual drugs, their dosages, and the schedule of their administration. Preexisting poor oral hygiene may also contribute to mucositis. Pain is often intense and interferes with oral intake. Chemotherapy-induced mucositis usually begins 3 to 5 days after therapy is started, reaches its peak at 7 to 10 days, and slowly resolves over the next 5 to 7 days unless complicated by infection or hemorrhage (Dreizen, 1990). Clinical signs of mucositis include diminished mucosal thickness and keratinization, superficial sloughing, and ulceration.

Radiation of the oropharyngeal and esophageal mucosa results in predictable inflammatory effects, usually appearing at the end of the second week of treatment, plateauing during the fourth week of radiation, and sometimes persisting for 2 to 3 weeks after the completion of treatment (Baker, 1982). Initially, the mucosa in the path of radiation

37

appears reddened and swollen; as treatment continues, the mucosa can be covered with a fibrous exudate.

In both chemotherapy- and radiation-associated mucositis pain, intensity is related to the extent of tissue damage and the degree of local inflammation. Typically, the patient describes a burning sensation, often accompanied by erythema. Because clinical signs and symptoms may change, patients with mucositis should be assessed frequently (Table 7). Management involves the aggressive use of analgesics (such as systemic patient-controlled analgesia) and agent-specific antimicrobial agents (Epstein, 1990; Janjan, Weissman, and Pahule, 1992).

Assessment of New Pain

Pain assessment is an ongoing process requiring constant attention to new pain (see Figure 1). **Changes in pain patterns or the development of new pain should not be attributed to preexisting causes but should instead trigger diagnostic evaluation.** New pain may signal treatable problems such as infection or fracture. A change in pain often signals advancing disease, and because pain management relies on the treatment of the underlying disease, establishing a medical diagnosis with the criteria discussed earlier is critical. A 1992 report showed that a comprehensive pain assessment revealed new causes of pain in 64 percent of 270 oncology patients with new pain complaints; most of the new diagnoses were neurologic (Gonzales, Payne, Foley, et al., 1992). Thus, the need to reassess persistent pain to identify new causes cannot be overemphasized.

3 Pharmacologic Management

Recommendations

13. An essential principle in using medications to manage cancer pain is to individualize the regimen to the patient. (A)

14. The simplest dosage schedules and least invasive pain management modalities should be used first. (Panel Consensus)

15. Pharmacologic management of mild to moderate cancer pain should include an NSAID or acetaminophen, unless there is a contraindication. (A)

16. When pain persists or increases, an opioid should be added. (A)

17. Treatment of persistent or moderate to severe pain should be based on increasing the opioid potency or dose. (A)

18. Medications for persistent cancer-related pain should be administered on an around-the-clock basis with additional "as-needed" doses, because regularly scheduled dosing maintains a constant level of drug in the body and helps to prevent a recurrence of pain. (A)

19. Patients receiving opioid agonists should not be given a mixed agonist-antagonist because doing so may precipitate a withdrawal syndrome and increase pain. (B)

20. Meperidine should not be used if continued opioid use is anticipated. (B)

21. Opioid tolerance and physical dependence are expected with long-term opioid treatment and should not be confused with addiction. (Panel Consensus)

22. The oral route is the preferred route of analgesic administration because it is the most convenient and cost-effective method of administration. When patients cannot take medications orally, rectal and transdermal routes should be considered because they are also relatively noninvasive. (Panel Consensus)

23. Intramuscular administration of drugs should be avoided because this route can be painful and inconvenient, and absorption is not reliable. (B)

24. Failure of maximal systemic doses of opioids and coanalgesics should precede the consideration of intraspinal analgesic systems. (Panel Consensus)

25. **Because there is great interindividual variation in susceptibility to opioid-induced side effects, clinicians should monitor for these potential side effects. (B)**

26. **Constipation is a common problem associated with long-term opioid administration and should be anticipated, treated prophylactically, and monitored constantly. (B)**

27. **Naloxone, when indicated for reversal of opioid-induced respiratory depression, should be titrated in doses that improve respiratory function but do not reverse analgesia. (B)**

28. **Placebos should not be used in the management of cancer pain. (Panel Consensus)**

29. **Patients should be given a written pain management plan. (A)**

30. **Communication about pain management should occur when a patient is transferred from one setting to another. (B)**

Drug therapy is the cornerstone of the many modalities available to manage cancer pain because it is effective, relatively low risk, inexpensive, and usually of rapid onset. **An essential principle in using medications to manage cancer pain is to individualize the regimen to the patient** (Foley, 1985a).

Three major classes of drugs are used alone or, more commonly, in combination to manage pain in the cancer patient:

■ NSAIDs and acetaminophen (APAP).

■ Opioid analgesics.

■ Adjuvant analgesics.

Before choosing drugs to manage pain or other symptoms, identify the specific cause(s) of the pain, evaluate its intensity and quality, and then match the drug to the pain intensity and other characteristics. **The simplest dosage schedules and least invasive pain management modalities should be used first.** After drug therapy has been started, pain should be assessed to determine the ongoing effectiveness of the analgesic therapy. For opioid analgesics, if pain relief is inadequate, the dose should be increased until pain relief is achieved or unacceptable side effects occur. In the case of NSAIDs and adjuvant analgesic drugs, which have ceiling effects to their analgesic efficacy, if the upper limit of the recommended dose is reached and pain relief is not achieved, then that particular drug should be discontinued and a second drug in that class should be used.

Most cancer pain can be managed by oral administration of drugs; however, difficulty in swallowing, gastrointestinal (GI) disturbances that render drug absorption unreliable, the amount of drug required, and many other factors may require alternative routes of administration (Coyle, Adelhardt, Foley, et al., 1990; Grond, Zech, Schug, et al., 1991). Table 8 summarizes some of the advantages and disadvantages of cancer pain therapies.

The WHO Ladder

A simple, well-validated, and effective method for assuring the rational titration of therapy for cancer pain has been devised by WHO (World Health Organization, 1990). It has been shown to be effective in relieving pain for approximately 90 percent of patients with cancer (Ventafridda, Caraceni, and Gamba, 1990) and over 75 percent of cancer patients who are terminally ill (Grond, Zech, Schug, et al., 1991). This approach is based on the concept of an analgesic ladder (Figure 2).

The five essential concepts in the WHO approach to drug therapy of cancer pain are:

- By the mouth.

- By the clock.

- By the ladder.

- For the individual.

- With attention to detail.

The first step in this approach is the use of acetaminophen, aspirin, or another NSAID for mild to moderate pain. Adjuvant drugs to enhance analgesic efficacy, treat concurrent symptoms that exacerbate pain, and provide independent analgesic activity for specific types of pain may be used at any step.

When pain persists or increases, an opioid such as codeine or hydrocodone should be added (not substituted) to the NSAID. Opioids at this step are often administered in fixed dose combinations with acetaminophen or aspirin because this combination provides additive analgesia (Weingart, Sorkness, and Earhart, 1985). Fixed-combination products may be limited by the content of acetaminophen or NSAID, which may produce dose-related toxicity. When higher doses of opioid are necessary, the third step is used. At this step separate dosage forms of the opioid and nonopioid analgesic should be used to avoid exceeding maximally recommended doses of acetaminophen or NSAID.

Pain that is persistent, or moderate to severe at the outset, should be treated by increasing opioid potency or using higher dosages.

continued on page 45

Table 8. Advantages and disadvantages of pain therapies

Intervention	Advantages	Disadvantages
Oral analgesics Acetaminophen Aspirin NSAIDs	1. Useful for a wide variety of mild to moderate pains. 2. Widely available, some over the counter. 3. Additive analgesia when combined with opioids and other modalities. 4. Can be administered by patient or family. 5. Some are inexpensive.	1. Ceiling effect to analgesia. 2. Side effects, especially gastritis and renal toxicity, can be serious. 3. May risk bleeding in severely thrombocytopenic patients. 4. Only one NSAID (ketorolac) is available now for parenteral administration. 5. Many are expensive.
Oral opioids	1. Effective for both localized and generalized pain. 2. Ceiling to analgesic effectiveness imposed only by side effects. 3. Multiple drug choices in this class. 4. Sedative and anxiolytic properties useful in some acute treatment settings. 5. Can be administered by patient or family. 6. Some are inexpensive. 7. Long acting, controlled-release forms available.	1. Side effects may limit analgesic effectiveness. 2. Prescription of these substances is regulated. 3. Stigma or fears associated with use.
Transdermal opioids (fentanyl)	1. Long duration of action (48–72 hours) from single patch. 2. Allows use of a strong opioid (fentanyl) in outpatient settings for some patients who have not tolerated morphine and related drugs. 3. Many patients find them easy to use. 4. Provides continuous administration of an opioid without use of needles or pumps. 5. Can be administered by patient or family.	1. Side effects may not be as quickly reversible as in oral opioid administration. 2. Difficult to modify dosage rapidly. 3. Relatively slow onset of action. 4. Requires additional short-acting medicine for breakthrough pain. 5. Expensive.
Rectal opioids	1. Relatively easy-to-use alternative route when the oral route is unavailable. 2. Other opioid suppositories available for morphine-intolerant patients. 3. Can be administered by patient or family. 4. Less expensive than subcutaneous or intravenous infusions.	1. Not widely accepted by patients or families. 2. Side effects may limit analgesic effectiveness. 3. Relatively slow onset of action. 4. Contraindicated if low white blood cell or platelet counts (risks of infection, bleeding).
Subcutaneous infusion	1. Can provide rapid pain relief without intravenous access. 2. Morphine or hydromorphone are the preferred drugs for this route when administered in the home. 3. When used in PCA mode, allows for rapid individual dose titration and provides sense of control for patient.	1. Only a limited volume of infusate can be administered (e.g., 2 to 4 ml/hour). 2. Induration, irritation at infusion site may be a complication. 3. Requires skilled nursing and pharmacy support. 4. Often requires expensive drug infusion pump and recurring charges for disposables.

Intervention	Advantages	Disadvantages
Intravenous infusion	1. Can provide rapid pain relief. 2. Almost all opioids can be given by this route. 3. Not limited by infusate volumes. 4. When used in PCA mode, allows for rapid individual dose titration and provides sense of control for patient.	1. Infection and infiltration of intravenous lines are potential complications. 2. Requires skilled nursing and pharmacy support. 3. Often requires expensive drug infusion pump and recurring charges for disposables.
Epidural, intrathecal, and intracerebral ventricular routes	1. Useful for pain that has not responded to less invasive measures. 2. Local anesthetics may be added to spinal opioids and may produce additive analgesia.	1. Tolerance may occur sooner than with oral or rectal administration. 2. Infection at catheter site can produce meningitis and/or epidural abscess. 3. Pruritus and urinary retention are more common than with oral or parenteral opioid administration. 4. Contraindicated in presence of acute spinal cord compression. 5. Requires special expertise. 6. Requires careful monitoring, especially when therapy begins and when doses are increased. 7. May require expensive drug infusion pump, intervention fees, and recurring charges for disposables.
Regional neurolytic blocks	1. Effective for pain relief with certain diagnoses (e.g., pancreatic cancer). 2. May be useful for movement-related and abdominal visceral pain that is refractory to drug therapy. 3. Can allow dosage (and side effect) reduction of systemic drugs for localized pain.	1. Risk of postural hypotension, bowel and bladder incontinence, and leg weakness. 2. Procedure is irreversible. 3. Requires special expertise. 4. Expenses for specialized care and operating room costs.
Ablative neurosurgery	1. May be useful for movement-related lower body pain that is refractory to drug therapy. 2. Fast onset of pain relief. 3. Percutaneous cordotomy can be done under local anesthesia. 4. Can allow dosage (and side effect) reduction of systemic drugs for localized pain.	1. Six-month duration of pain relief for cordotomy is only 50%. 2. Procedure is irreversible. 3. Requires special expertise. 4. Expensive because of specialized care and operating room costs.

Table 8. Advantages and disadvantages of pain therapies, continued

Intervention	Advantages	Disadvantages
Corticosteroids	1. Effective in pain associated with inflammatory component (e.g., bone pain). 2. Can produce cytotoxic effect against some tumors. 3. May be given orally or intravenously. 4. May increase appetite. 5. May produce euphoria in some patients. 6. May decrease pain associated with CNS and spinal cord tumors.	1. Prolonged use associated with adrenal suppression, fluid and electrolyte disturbance. 2. Increases risk of gastritis. 3. Prolonged use may decrease cell-mediated immunity and increase risk of infection. 4. Some patients experience emotional instability or psychoses. 5. May suppress (mask) fevers associated with infections.
Anticonvulsants	1. Useful for peripheral pain syndromes associated with neuropathic pain, especially lancinating or shooting pain.	1. May increase sedation. 2. Monitoring required to avoid specific toxicities associated with increased serum levels. 3. Idiosyncratic or dose-related bone marrow suppression may limit usefulness.
Antidepressants	1. Useful in pain syndromes associated with neuropathic pain and with pain caused by surgery, chemotherapy, or nerve infiltration. 2. May promote sleep when taken at bedtime.	1. May increase sedation. 2. Anticholinergic side effects of many antidepressants are distressing to many patients. 3. CNS, cardiovascular, and hepatic toxicities may limit usefulness.
Hydroxyzine	1. When given in high dosages (100 mg),some antihistamines may produce additive analgesia with therapeutic doses of opioids. 2. May be beneficial in patients with opioid-induced nausea and vomiting.	1. In high doses demonstrates a significant potential for causing respiratory depression which is additive to that of opioids, but not reversible with naloxone. 2. Can cause significant sedation.
Radiation therapy	1. Directly treats tumor, especially useful for bone metastasis. 2. Can provide fast onset of pain relief. 3. Single dose is effective for some patients. 4. Widely available mode of treatment. 5. Radiopharmaceuticals and some forms of radiation therapy can treat multiple disease sites.	1. When multiple fractions are given, it may entail prolonged inconvenience and discomfort for patients. 2. Myelosuppression may occur, especially with prior chemotherapy when wide teletherapy or radiopharmaceuticals are used.
Relaxation, imagery, biofeedback, distraction, and reframing	1. May decrease pain and anxiety without drug-related side effects. 2. Can be used as adjuvant therapy with most other modalities. 3. Can increase patient's sense of control. 4. Most are inexpensive, require no special equipment, and are easily administered.	1. Patient must be motivated to use self-management strategies. 2. Requires professional time to teach interventions.

Intervention	Advantages	Disadvantages
Patient education	1. Effective in improving ability to follow medical regimen and in decreasing pain. 2. Multiple teaching aids available. 3. Promotes self-care in pain treatment and management of side effects.	1. Requires professional time to teach pain management regimens.
Psychotherapy, structured support, and hypnosis	1. May decrease pain and anxiety for patients who have pain that is difficult to manage. 2. May increase patient's coping skills.	1. Requires skilled therapist.
Cutaneous stimulation (superficial heat, cold, and massage)	1. May reduce pain, inflammation, and/or muscle spasm. 2. Can be used as adjuvant therapy with most other modalities. 3. Relatively easy to use. 4. Can be administered by patients or families. 5. Relatively low cost.	1. Heat may increase bleeding and edema after acute injury. 2. Cold is contraindicated for use over ischemic tissues.
Transcutaneous electrical nerve stimulation	1. May provide pain relief without drug-related side effects. 2. Can be used as adjuvant therapy with most other modalities. 3. Gives patient sense of control over pain.	1. Requires skilled therapist to initiate therapy. 2. Potential risk of infection, bleeding.
Acupuncture	1. May provide pain relief without side effects. 2. Can be used as adjuvant with most other therapies.	1. Requires skilled therapist.
Peer support groups	1. May increase patient's coping skills. 2. Increases sense of control. 3. Provides support for families and patients.	1. None identified.
Pastoral counseling	1. May increase patient's coping skills. 2. May provide spiritual and emotional comfort.	1. None identified.

Drugs such as codeine or hydrocodone are replaced with more potent opioids (usually morphine, hydromorphone, methadone, fentanyl, or levorphanol), as described below.

Medications for persistent cancer-related pain should be administered on an around-the-clock basis, with additional "as-needed" doses, because regularly scheduled dosing maintains a constant level of drug in the body and helps to prevent a recurrence of pain. Patients who have moderate to severe pain when first seen by the clinician should be started at the second or third step of the ladder.

Nonsteroidal Anti-Inflammatory Drugs (NSAIDs)

NSAIDs are used as initial therapy in mild pain because they are effective, are often available over the counter, and can be used effectively in combination with opioids and adjuvant analgesics if pain intensity increases. Acetaminophen is included with this group, even though its anti-inflammatory effects are less potent, because it has similar analgesic potency and pharmacologic characteristics. A major advantage of acetaminophen in comparison to other NSAIDs is its lack of effect on platelet function, which makes it less risky to use in thrombocytopenic patients. It is also relatively inexpensive.

NSAIDs decrease levels of inflammatory mediators generated at the site of tissue injury by inhibiting the enzyme cyclooxygenase, which catalyzes the conversion of arachidonic acid to prostaglandins and leukotrienes (Sunshine and Olson, 1989). These mediators sensitize nerves to painful stimuli. Although NSAIDs may also affect the central nervous system, these drugs do not activate opioid receptors and therefore produce analgesia by a different mechanism than opioids. Hence:

- The concurrent use of opioids, NSAIDs, and acetaminophen often provides more analgesia than does either of the drug classes alone.

- The addition of NSAIDs and acetaminophen to opioid analgesics may achieve a "dose-sparing" effect such that lower doses of opioids may now produce pain relief with fewer side effects (Hodsman, Burns, Blyth, et al., 1987; Weingart, Sorkness, and Earhart, 1985).

In contrast to opioids, NSAIDs do not produce tolerance, physical, or psychological dependence, are antipyretic, and have a different spectrum of toxicity. Used as single agents, NSAIDs have a ceiling effect on their analgesic potential, so the use of doses higher than those specified in the package insert is not recommended.

The nonacetylated salicylates such as salsalate, sodium salicylate, and choline magnesium trisalicylate do not affect platelet aggregation profoundly and do not alter bleeding time (Danesh, Saniabadi, Russell, et al., 1987; Day, Furst, Graham, et al., 1987; Estes and Kaplan, 1980; Morris, Sherman, McQuain, et al., 1985; Stuart and Pisko, 1981; Zucker and Rothwell, 1978). Aspirin, the prototype of the acetylated salicylate, produces an irreversible inhibition of platelet aggregation, which may prolong bleeding time for up to several days after ingestion (Stuart, Murphy, Oski, et al., 1972; Sutor, Bowie, and Owen, 1971; Weiss, Aledont, and Kochwa, 1968). The nonacetylated salicylates, such as sodium salicylate and choline magnesium trisalicylate, have minimal effects on platelet aggregation and do not appear to alter bleeding time clinically (Day, Furst, Graham, et al., 1987; Morris, Sherman, McQuain, et al., 1985; Stuart and Pisko, 1981; Zucker and Rothwell, 1978). Other NSAIDs produce a reversible inhibition of platelet aggregation, which persists while the drug is in the systemic circulation (Schlegel, 1987). Therefore, with the exception of the nonacetylated salicylates noted above, NSAIDs should be avoided if possible in patients who are thrombocytopenic or who have a clotting impairment.

NSAIDs bind extensively to plasma proteins and therefore may be displaced by or may displace other protein-bound drugs such as coumadin, methotrexate, digoxin, cyclosporine, oral antidiabetic agents, and sulfa drugs. Such interactions may enhance therapeutic or toxic effects of either drug. The use of NSAIDs has been associated with both minor (dyspepsia, heartburn, nausea, vomiting, anorexia, diarrhea, constipation, flatulence, bloating, epigastric pain, and abdominal pain) and major (bleeding, ulceration, and perforation) GI toxicities. Serious effects are not always preceded by minor GI effects; patients should be advised to report any GI disturbances.

Hepatic and renal dysfunction or toxicity, which can occur at any time in the course of NSAID therapy, are of particular concern during long-term use (Sunshine and Olson, 1989). The risk of renal dysfunction is greatest in patients with advanced age, preexisting renal impairment, heart failure, hepatic dysfunction, hypovolemia, concomitant therapy with other nephrotoxic drugs such as diuretics, or elevated levels of angiotensin II or catecholamines. Antipyretic and anti-inflammatory effects of NSAIDs may mask the usual signs and symptoms of infections.

Adverse effects of NSAIDs that may appear at any time include:

■ **Renal failure.**

■ **Hepatic dysfunction.**

■ **Bleeding.**

■ **Gastric ulceration.**

Even though NSAIDs are effective in relieving mild pain and are opioid sparing for moderate to severe pain, patients who take them, especially if elderly, should be monitored carefully for adverse effects.

Most NSAIDs are available as oral tablets, caplets, or capsules, and several are available as oral liquids. Rectal suppositories of aspirin, acetaminophen, and other NSAIDs are commercially available or can be compounded easily by pharmacists. Ketorolac tromethamine is the only NSAID that is currently available for short-term parenteral administration. Table 9 provides dosing data for acetaminophen and NSAIDs.

Table 9. Dosing data for acetaminophen (APAP) and NSAIDs

Drug	Usual dose for adults and children $\geq$ 50 kg body weight	Usual dose for children[1] and adults[2] $\leq$ 50 kg body weight
Acetaminophen and over-the-counter NSAIDs		
Acetaminophen[3]	650 mg q 4 h 975 mg q 6 h	10-15 mg/kg q 4 h 15-20 mg/kg q 4 h (rectal)
Aspirin[4]	650 mg q 4 h 975 mg q 6 h	10-15 mg/kg q 4 h 15-20 mg/kg q 4 h (rectal)
Ibuprofen (Motrin, others)	400-600 mg q 6 h	10 mg/kg q 6–8 h[5]
Prescription NSAIDs		
Carprofen (Rimadyl)	100 mg tid	
Choline magnesium trisalicylate[6] (Trilisate)	1,000-1,500 mg tid	25 mg/kg tid
Choline salicylate (Arthropan)[6]	870 mg q 3-4 h	
Diflunisal (Dolobid)[7]	500 mg q 12 h	
Etodolac (Lodine)	200-400 mg q 6-8 h	
Fenoprofen calcium (Nalfon)	300-600 mg q 6 h	
Ketoprofen (Orudis)	25-60 mg q 6-8 h	
Ketorolac tromethamine[8] (Toradol)	10 mg q 4-6 h to a maximum of 40 mg/day	
Magnesium salicylate (Doan's, Magan, Mobidin, others)	650 mg q 4 h	
Meclofenamate sodium (Meclomen)[9]	50-100 mg q 6 h	
Mefenamic acid (Ponstel)	250 mg q 6 h	
Naproxen (Naprosyn)	250-275 mg q 6-8 h	5 mg/kg q 8 h
Naproxen sodium (Anaprox)	275 mg q 6-8 h	
Sodium salicylate (Generic)	325-650 mg q 3-4 h	
Parenteral NSAIDs		
Ketorolac tromethamine[8, 10] (Toradol)	60 mg initially, then 30 mg q 6 h Intramuscular dose not to exceed 5 days	

48

It is impossible to predict which NSAID will be best tolerated by a particular patient; no particular NSAID has demonstrated superiority over others for pain relief. Once an NSAID has been selected, the dose should be increased until pain has been relieved or the maximal recommended dose has been achieved. The duration of analgesia does not always correlate with the serum half-life of the NSAID. Therefore, the response of the patient should guide the clinician in selecting dosing intervals of these agents. Because NSAIDs and adjuvant analgesics have ceiling effects to their efficacy, if a patient does not respond to the maximal dose of one NSAID, another should be tried before discontinuation of NSAID therapy. The initial choice of NSAID should be based on the efficacy, safety, and relative expense; generally, the least expensive NSAID should be chosen.

Opioids

Opioids are the major class of analgesics used in the management of moderate to severe pain because of their effectiveness, ease of titration, and favorable risk-to-benefit ratio. Opioids produce analgesia by binding to specific receptors both within and outside the CNS (Stein, 1993; Hargreaves and Joris, 1993). Opioid analgesics are classified as full agonists, partial agonists, or mixed agonist-antagonists, depending on the specific receptors to which they bind and their intrinsic activity at that receptor.

Commonly used full agonists include morphine, hydromorphone, codeine, oxycodone, hydrocodone, methadone, levorphanol, and fentanyl. These opioids are classified as full agonists because they do not have a ceiling to their analgesic efficacy and will not reverse or

---

[1] Only drugs that are FDA approved as an analgesic for use in children are included.

[2] Acetaminophen and NSAID dosages for adults weighing less than 50 kg should be adjusted for weight.

[3] APAP lacks the peripheral anti-inflammatory and antiplatelet activities of the other NSAIDs.

[4] The standard against which other NSAIDs are compared. May inhibit platelet aggregation for ≥1 week and may cause bleeding. Aspirin is contraindicated in children with fever or other viral disease because of its association with Reye's syndrome.

[5] Not FDA approved for use in children as an over-the-counter drug; has FDA approval for use in children as a prescription drug for fever. However, clinicians have experience in prescribing ibuprofen for pain in children.

[6] May have minimal antiplatelet activity.

[7] Administration with antacids may decrease absorption.

[8] For short-term use only.

[9] Coombs-positive autoimmune hemolytic anemia has been associated with prolonged use.

[10] Has the same GI toxicities as oral NSAIDs.

Note: Only the above NSAIDs have FDA approval for use as simple analgesics, but clinical experience has been gained with other drugs as well.

antagonize the effects of other opioids within this class given simultaneously. Side effects include constipation, nausea, urinary retention, confusion, sedation, and respiratory depression.

Buprenorphine is a partial agonist. It has a relatively low intrinsic efficacy at the opioid receptor in comparison to full opioid agonists and displays a ceiling effect to analgesia.

Mixed agonist-antagonists in clinical use include pentazocine, butorphanol tartrate, dezocine, and nalbuphine hydrochloride. These drugs have an analgesic ceiling. In contrast to full agonists, these drugs block opioid analgesia at one type of opioid receptor (mu) or are neutral at this receptor while simultaneously activating a different opioid receptor (kappa). **Patients receiving full opioid agonists should not be given a mixed agonist-antagonist because doing so may precipitate a withdrawal syndrome and increase pain.**

Morphine is the most commonly used opioid for moderate to severe pain because of its availability in a wide variety of dosage forms, its well-characterized pharmacokinetics and pharmacodynamics, and its relatively low cost.

Meperidine may be useful for brief courses (e.g., a few days) to treat acute pain and to manage rigors (shivering) induced by medication, but it generally should be avoided in patients with cancer because of its short duration of action (2.5 to 3.5 hours) and its toxic metabolite, normeperidine. This metabolite accumulates, particularly when renal function is impaired, and causes CNS stimulation, which may lead to dysphoria, agitation, and seizures (Kaiko, Foley, Grabinski, et al., 1983). **Therefore, meperidine should not be used if continued opioid use is anticipated.**

Equianalgesic doses of commonly used opioids and starting doses for those drugs are listed in Tables 10 and 11.

Tolerance and Physical Dependence

Opioid tolerance and physical dependence are expected with long-term opioid treatment and should not be confused with psychological dependence ("addiction"), manifested as drug abuse behavior. The misunderstanding of these terms in relation to opioid use leads to ineffective practices in prescribing, administering, and dispensing opioids for cancer pain and contributes to the problem of undertreatment.

The presence of opioid tolerance and physical dependence does not equate with "addiction."

Physical dependence on opioids is revealed when the opioid is abruptly discontinued or when naloxone is administered and is typically manifested as anxiety, irritability, chills and hot flashes, joint pain, lacrimation, rhinorrhea, diaphoresis, nausea, vomiting, and abdominal cramps and diarrhea. The mildest form of the opioid abstinence syndrome may be confused with viral "flu-like" syndromes. For opioids with short half-lives (i.e., codeine, hydrocodone, morphine, hydromorphone), the onset of withdrawal symptoms can occur within 6 to 12 hours and peak at 24 to 72 hours after discontinuation. For opioids with long half-lives (i.e., methadone, levorphanol, transdermal fentanyl), the onset of the abstinence syndrome may be delayed for 24 hours or more after drug discontinuation and may be of milder intensity. The appearance of the abstinence syndrome defines physical dependence on opioids, which may occur after just 2 weeks of opioid therapy, but does not imply psychological dependence or addiction. Most patients with cancer take opioids for more than 2 weeks, and only very rarely do they exhibit the drug abuse behaviors and psychological dependence that characterize addiction (Portenoy and Payne, 1992).

Patients with cancer occasionally require discontinuation or rapid decreases in doses of opioids when the cause of pain is effectively eliminated by antineoplastic treatments or pain perception is modified by neuroablative or neurolytic procedures. In such circumstances, the opioid abstinence syndrome can be avoided by withdrawal of the opioid on a schedule that provides half the prior daily dose for each of the first 2 days and then reduces the daily dose by 25 percent every 2 days thereafter until the total dose (in morphine equivalents) is 30 mg/day. The drug may be discontinued after 2 days on the 30 mg/day dose (American Pain Society, 1992). Transdermal clonidine (0.1 to 0.2 mg/day) may reduce anxiety, tachycardia, and other autonomic symptoms associated with opioid withdrawal.

Tolerance to opioids is defined as the need to increase dose requirements over time to maintain pain relief. For most cancer patients, the first indication of tolerance is a decrease in the duration of analgesia for a given dose. Increasing dose requirements are most consistently correlated with progressive disease, which produces increased pain intensity (Foley, 1985a). Patients with stable disease do not usually require increasing doses (Foley, 1993; Levy, 1989).

Dosage Titration

Opioid doses should be adjusted in each patient to achieve pain relief with an acceptable level of adverse effects. Dosage typically requires adjustment over time. With the exception of fentanyl delivered by the transdermal route, there is no ceiling or maximal recommended dose for full opioid agonists, and in fact, very large doses of morphine, e.g., several hundred milligrams every 4 hours, may be needed for severe pain (Foley, 1985a).

Effective pain relief can be accomplished by the anticipation and prevention of pain. **Because many patients have persistent or daily**

Table 10. Dose equivalents for opioid analgesics in opioid-naive adults and children ⩾50 kg body weight[1]

Drug	Approximate equianalgesic dose		Usual starting dose for moderate to severe pain	
	Oral	Parenteral	Oral	Parenteral
Opioid agonist[2]				
Morphine[3]	30 mg q 3-4 h (repeat around-the-clock dosing) 60 mg q 3-4 h (single dose or intermittent dosing)	10 mg q 3-4 h	30 mg q 3-4 h	10 mg q 3-4 h
Morphine, controlled-release[3,4] (MS Contin, Oramorph)	90-120 mg q 12 h	N/A	90-120 mg q 12 h	N/A
Hydromorphone[3] (Dilaudid)	7.5 mg q 3-4 h	1.5 mg q 3-4 h	6 mg q 3-4 h	1.5 mg q 3-4 h
Levorphanol (Levo-Dromoran)	4 mg q 6-8 h	2 mg q 6-8 h	4 mg q 6-8 h	2 mg q 6-8 h
Meperidine (Demerol)	300 mg q 2-3 h	100 mg q 3 h	N/R	100 mg q 3 h
Methadone (Dolophine, other)	20 mg q 6-8 h	10 mg q 6-8 h	20 mg q 6-8 h	10 mg q 6-8 h
Oxymorphone[3] (Numorphan)	N/A	1 mg q 3-4 h	N/A	1 mg q 3-4 h
Combination opioid/NSAID preparations[5]				
Codeine[6] (with aspirin or acetaminophen)	180-200 mg q 3-4 h	130 mg q 3-4 h	60 mg q 3-4 h	60 mg q 2 h (IM/SC)
Hydrocodone (in Lorcet, Lortab, Vicodin, others)	30 mg q 3-4 h	N/A	10 mg q 3-4 h	N/A
Oxycodone (Roxicodone, also in Percocet, Percodan, Tylox, others)	30 mg q 3-4 h	N/A	10 mg q 3-4 h	N/A

[1] Caution: Recommended doses do not apply for adult patients with body weight less than 50 kg. For recommended starting doses for children and adults < 50 kg body weight, see Table 11.
[2] Caution: Recommended doses do not apply to patients with renal or hepatic insufficiency or other conditions affecting drug metabolism and kinetics.
[3] Caution: For morphine, hydromorphone, and oxymorphone, rectal administration is an alternate route for patients unable to take oral medications. Equianalgesic doses may differ from

52

pain, it is important to use opioids on a regular schedule rather than only "as needed." Around-the-clock administration of analgesics allows each dose to become effective before the previous dose has lost its effectiveness. A patient should be given "as-needed" doses for the first 24 to 48 hours when a new drug is started to define the best daily dosing requirements for that individual patient.

In addition to the titration of individual drugs, the modalities for pain management are titrated when the pain is persistent and is moderate to severe in intensity (see Figure 3).

Pain management for moderate to severe pain should begin with oral opioids in combination with an NSAID or acetaminophen. The optimal dose will control pain with the fewest side effects, such as sedation, mental clouding, nausea, or constipation.

Adjuvant drugs (see below) may be used to counteract the predictable side effects of opioids. For example, hydroxyzine may be added to opioids and NSAIDs to manage anxiety and nausea, especially when they occur simultaneously and are not intense. Dietary caffeine supplementation may provide additive analgesia and counteract opioid induced sedation. Antiemetic drugs such as phenothiazines and metoclopramide may be added to manage opioid-induced nausea.

It is usually advisable to observe the patient's response to several different opioids, sequentially, before switching routes of administration or trying an anesthetic, neurosurgical, or other invasive approach to relieve persistent pain (Galer, Coyle, Pasternak, et al., 1992). For example, patients who experience dose-limiting sedation, nausea, or mental clouding on oral morphine should be switched to an equianalgesic dose of hydromorphone or fentanyl. The dose of the second opioid should then be adjusted. Sequential analgesic trials should be based on regular

---

oral and parenteral doses because of pharmacokinetic differences.

[4]Transdermal fentanyl (Duragesic) is an alternative option. Transdermal fentanyl dosage is not calculated as equianalgesic to a single morphine dose. See the package insert for dosing calculations. Doses above 25 μg/h should not be used in opiod-naive patients.

[5]Caution: Doses of aspirin and acetaminophen in combination opioid/NSAID preparations must also be adjusted to the patient's body weight. Aspirin is contraindicated in children in the presence of fever or other viral disease because of its association with Reye's syndrome.

[6]Caution: Codeine doses above 65 mg often are not appropriate because of diminishing incremental analgesia with increasing doses but continually increasing nausea, constipation, and other side effects.

Note: Published tables vary in the suggested doses that are equianalgesic to morphine. Clinical response is the criterion that must be applied for each patient; titration to clinical responses is necessary. Because there is not complete cross-tolerance among these drugs, it is usually necessary to use a lower than equianalgesic dose when changing drugs and to retitrate to response.

Codes: q=every. N/A=not available. N/R=not recommended. IM=intramuscular. SC=subcutaneous.

Table 11. Dose equivalent for opioid analgesics in opioid-naive children and adults <50 kg body weight[1]

Drug	Approximate equianalgesic dose		Usual starting dose for moderate to severe pain	
	Oral	Parenteral	Oral	Parenteral
Opioid agonist[2]				
Morphine[3]	30 mg q 3-4 h (repeat around-the-clock dosing) 60 mg q 3-4 h (single dose or intermittent dosing)	10 mg q 3-4 h	0.3 mg/kg q 3-4 h	0.1 mg/kg q 3-4 h
Morphine controlled-release[3,4] (MS Contin, Oramorph)	90-120 mg q 12 h	N/A	N/A	N/A
Hydromorphone[3] (Dilaudid)	7.5 mg q 3-4 h	1.5 mg q 3-4 h	0.06 mg/kg q 3-4 h	0.015 mg/kg q 3-4 h
Levorphanol (Levo-Dromoran)	4 mg q 6-8 h	2 mg q 6-8 h	0.04 mg/kg q 6-8 h	0.02 mg/kg q 6-8 h
Meperidine (Demerol)	300 mg q 2-3 h	100 mg q 3 h	N/R	0.75 mg/kg q 2-3 h
Methadone (Dolophine, others)	20 mg q 6-8 h	10 mg q 6-8 h	0.2 mg/kg q 6-8 h	0.1 mg/kg q 6-8 h
Combination opioid/NSAID preparations[5]				
Codeine[6] (with aspirin or acetaminophen)	180-200 mg q 3-4 h	130 mg q 3-4 h	0.5-1 mg/kg q 3-4 h	N/R
Hydrocodone (in Lorcet, Lortab, Vicodin, others)	30 mg q 3-4 h	N/A	0.2 mg/kg q 3-4 h	N/A
Oxycodone (Roxicodone, also in Percocet, Percodan, Tylox, others)	30 mg q 3-4 h	N/A	0.2 mg/kg q 3-4 h	N/A

[1]Caution: Doses listed for patients with body weight less than 50 kg cannot be used as initial starting doses in babies less than 6 months of age.

[2]Caution: Recommended doses do not apply to patients with renal or hepatic insufficiency or other conditions affecting drug metabolism and kinetics.

[3]Caution: For morphine, hydromorphone, and oxymorphone, rectal administration is an alternate route for patients unable to take oral medications. Equianalgesic doses may differ from oral and parenteral doses because of pharmacokinetic differences.

[4]Transdermal fentanyl (Duragesic) is an alternative option. Transdermal fentanyl dosage is not calculated as equianalgesic to a single morphine dosage. See the package insert for dosing

54

assessments of pain, with continuous attention to antineoplastic and noninvasive nonpharmacologic therapies (see Figure 1).

Administration Methods

The speed of onset and duration of action for any opioid depend on the specific drug chosen and its formulation (tablet, elixir, etc.). Most are well absorbed after oral or rectal administration, yet absorption may not be complete. Further, drugs absorbed from the gut are subject to first-pass metabolism in the liver and, hence, should be given at higher doses than when given parenterally. Although dosage requirements for different parenteral routes (intravenous, subcutaneous, and intramuscular) are comparable or equivalent, the onset of drug action is typically most rapid after intravenous dosing because there is no delay in absorption. Therefore, drug dose and frequency should be titrated to the individual patient's response and analgesic needs when changing the route of administration or the type of formulation.

Oral. The oral route is the preferred route of analgesic administration because it is the most convenient and cost-effective. Oral opioids are available in tablet, capsule, and liquid forms and in immediate and controlled-release formulations; morphine is available in immediate and controlled-release forms. Controlled-release tablets become immediately released when crushed and are therefore not appropriate for patients who are unable to swallow whole tablets. A small percentage may require alternate routes during their illness and when they are unable to swallow, such as during mucositis or in the terminal phase. Coyle, Adelhardt, Foley, et al. (1990) found that many patients required more than one route of administration to maintain pain control in the last 4 weeks of life. **When patients cannot take medications orally, other less invasive routes such as rectal or transdermal routes should be tried.** During intravenous and subcutaneous administration, local irritation of the skin or vein may occur. Therefore,

---

calculations. Doses above 25 μg/h should not be used in opioid-naive patients.
[5]Caution: Doses of aspirin and acetaminophen in combination opioid/NSAID preparations must also be adjusted to the patient's body weight. Aspirin is contraindicated in children in the presence of fever or other viral disease because of its association with Reye's syndrome.
[6]Caution: Some clinicians recommend not exceeding 1.5 mg/kg of codeine because of an increased incidence of side effects with higher doses.

Note: Published tables vary in the suggested doses that are equianalgesic to morphine. Clinical response is the criterion that must be applied for each patient; titration to clinical responses is necessary. Because there is not complete cross-tolerance among these drugs, it is usually necessary to use a lower than equianalgesic dose when changing drugs and to retitrate to response.

Codes: q=every. N/A=not available. N/R=not recommended.

parenteral routes should be used only when simpler, less demanding, and less costly methods are inappropriate or ineffective.

Rectal. The rectal route may be used when patients have nausea or vomiting or are fasting either preoperatively or postoperatively. The rectal route is contraindicated if there are lesions of the anus or rectum because placement of the suppository will cause pain. This route is also not useful if there is diarrhea or in elderly or infirm patients who are physically unable to place the suppository.

There are commercially available suppositories of morphine, hydromorphone, and oxymorphone. Medications can also be placed in a colostomy or similar stoma, provided that the flow of effluent is slow enough to allow the drug to be absorbed via the mucosa (McCaffery, Martin, and Ferrell, 1992). When converting from the oral to the rectal route, start with the same amount as the oral dose and titrate as needed.

Transdermal. Transdermal administration bypasses GI absorption. Fentanyl is currently the only opioid commercially available in a transdermal form (TDS-Fentanyl). Four patch sizes are available and provide delivery of fentanyl at 25, 50, 75, or 100 μg/hour; therefore, there is flexibility in drug dosing. The maximal recommended daily dose is 300 μg/hour. Patients requiring larger doses should be switched to an equianalgesic dose of an oral or subcutaneously administered opioid.

Each patch contains a 72-hour supply of fentanyl, which is passively absorbed through the skin over this period. Levels in plasma rise slowly over 12 to 18 hours after patch placement, and the dosage form has an elimination half-life of 21 hours. Therefore, unlike intravenous fentanyl, the transdermal administration of fentanyl is not suitable for rapid dose titration (Payne, 1992; Portenoy, Southam, Gupta, et al., 1993). Transdermal fentanyl should be considered when patients already on opioid therapy have relatively constant pain and infrequent episodes of breakthrough pain such that rapid increases or decreases in pain intensity are not anticipated. As with other long acting analgesics, all patients should be provided with oral or parenteral rapidly acting short duration opioids to manage breakthrough pain (Portenoy and Hagen, 1990). The most commonly reported side effects of transdermal fentanyl administration are nausea, mental clouding, and skin irritation.

Nasal. The transnasal route is an alternative delivery method that may be useful when patients are no longer able to tolerate the oral route. Although several agents are currently being studied, the only commercially available formulation is the mixed agonist-antagonist drug butorphanol, which is rapidly taken up by the vascular nasal mucosa. The major indication for its use is acute headache. Although this formulation has general appeal by virtue of its potential for rapid action because it is a mixed agonist-antagonist, this drug is not recommended for routine use in cancer pain treatment.

Intravenous or Subcutaneous. **Intramuscular administration of drugs should be avoided because this route can be painful and inconvenient, and absorption is not reliable.** Intravenous or subcutaneous administration are effective alternatives. Patients who may benefit from continuous infusions of opioids include:

■ Those with persistent nausea and vomiting.

■ Those with severe dysphagia or swallowing disorders.

■ Those with delirium, confusion, stupor, or other mental status changes that make oral administration contraindicated because of concerns about pulmonary aspiration in an unprotected airway.

■ Those on high doses of oral medications necessitating numerous tablets.

■ Those who experience undesirable side effects in relation to each dose of an "as-needed" medication.

■ Those who require rapid incremental doses of analgesia.

The benefits of opioid infusions, compared with those of intermittent "as-needed" doses by intramuscular or subcutaneous injection, include less pain on injection, fewer delays awaiting preparation and administration of medication, and improved effectiveness (Bruera, Brenneis, and MacDonald, 1987; Portenoy, 1986, 1987). The intravenous route provides the most rapid onset of analgesia, but the duration of analgesia after a bolus dose is shorter than with other routes.

A continuous intravenous infusion provides the most consistent level of analgesia and is easily accomplished for patients who have permanent intravenous access for other purposes such as hydration, alimentation, chemotherapy, or antibiotic administration. If intravenous access is not available or desirable, continuous subcutaneous opioid infusion offers a practical alternative in the hospital and home. The subcutaneous administration of opioids provides levels in blood comparable to those with intravenous doses; therefore, the intravenous dose recommendations can be used (Tables 10 and 11) (Moulin, Kreeft, Murray-Parsons, et al., 1991).

Intraspinal. Analgesics may be administered intraspinally when pain cannot be controlled by oral, transdermal, subcutaneous, or intravenous routes because side effects such as confusion and nausea limit further dose escalation. **Documentation of the failure of maximal doses of opioids and coanalgesics administered through other routes should precede consideration of intraspinal analgesia.** Furthermore, this route requires experience, meticulous technique, significant family and professional support systems, and sophisticated followup, which are not available in all settings. Before implantation of a permanent device, screening should be conducted to ensure adequate response to spinal therapy. A trial of graded opioid doses administered percutaneously through an epidural catheter generally will indicate whether intraspinal therapy is warranted.

As with systemic opioid administration, the dose range for intraspinal opioid therapy varies widely, depending on the level of pain and tolerance (Du Pen and Williams, 1992). Any agent delivered into the epidural or intrathecal space should be free of preservatives because some preservatives and antioxidants can produce neurotoxicity when used intraspinally (Du Pen, Ramsey, and Chin, 1987; Wang, Hillman, Spielholz, et al., 1984). All patients treated with intraspinal drugs should have access to rescue medications (oral or parenteral) for periods of breakthrough pain or in the case of catheter or drug delivery system malfunction. The coadministration of systemic opioids (which generally is not recommended for postoperative pain management) is safe in most cancer patients because they are tolerant to the respiratory-depressant effects of the drugs.

Morphine is the most commonly used intraspinal drug. Alternative opioids such as hydromorphone, fentanyl, or sufentanil have been used intraspinally to manage cancer pain and may be useful substitutes when the patient experiences side effects from morphine. Intraspinal morphine may produce the same side effects of nausea, mental clouding, and sedation as in oral, rectal, or parenteral dosing, because epidural or subarachnoid morphine is absorbed into the circulation by way of the rich epidural vascular plexus and is also carried in the normal flow of cerebrospinal fluid (CSF) from spinal levels to the brain (Bromage, Camporesi, Durant, et al., 1982; Chauvin, Samii, Schermann, et al., 1982; Cousins, 1988; Max, Inturrisi, Kaiko, et al., 1985). Single-dose epidural administration of 10 mg of morphine produces levels in blood comparable to an intramuscular injection of the same dose (Max, Inturrisi, Kaiko, et al., 1985). Very lipophilic opioids such as fentanyl and sufentanil have a more limited CSF distribution, but these drugs also gain access to the blood and are delivered to the brain via the systemic circulation.

In some patients, it is possible to give relatively small doses of opioid spinally and produce pain relief while avoiding the side effects that can limit prior oral or parenteral dosing. However, patients with a high degree of tolerance to systemic opioids may require large doses of spinal opioids (Cousins and Bridenbaugh, 1987), which may negate the advantages of this targeted approach because side effects may still be prominent at high dosage levels.

The main indication for the long-term administration of intraspinal opioids is intractable pain in the lower part of the body, particularly when pain is bilateral or midline (Du Pen and Williams, 1992). With proper selection and screening, good to excellent pain relief can be expected in up to 90 percent of patients (Krames, Gershow, Glassberg, et al., 1985; Onofrio and Yaksh, 1990). Opioids (sometimes coadministered with other agents such as dilute local anesthetic) (Akerman, Arweström, and Post, 1988; Fraser, Chapman, and Dickenson, 1992; Maves and Gebhart, 1992; Tejwani, Rattan, and McDonald, 1992) are delivered to the epidural or subarachnoid space via percutaneously placed catheters connected to ports, reservoirs, or infusion pumps (Table 12). For short-term treatment of weeks to a few months, externalized catheters (tunneled or untunneled) can be used. For more prolonged treatment, the delivery system (catheter plus port or pump) can be internalized. Adverse sequelae include the development of tolerance, urinary retention, constipation, pruritus, device failure, and infection (Du Pen, Peterson, Williams, et al., 1990; Hogan, Haddox, Abram, et al., 1991).

Intraventricular. Experience with intraventricular morphine administration is steadily increasing, and results with this route compare favorably with those with intraspinal administration, with over 90 percent of patients in published series benefitting significantly (Choi, Ha, Ahn, et al., 1989). Most important, intraventricular morphine is beneficial for recalcitrant pain due to head and neck malignancies and tumors (e.g., superior sulcus tumors, breast carcinoma) that affect the brachial plexus. Small maintenance doses of morphine (less than 5 mg daily) are needed to achieve maximal comfort. Complications are rare, the most important being infection; as with intraspinal drug delivery, tolerance and respiratory depression do not appear to be major issues (Acute Pain Management Guideline Panel, 1992). Intraventricular morphine requires the placement of a ventricular catheter connected to a subcutaneous (e.g., Ommaya) reservoir for intermittent administration or an infusion pump for continuous infusion (Lazorthes, Verdie, Bastide, et al., 1985; Obbens, Hill, Leavens, et al., 1987).

Patient-Controlled Analgesia (PCA). PCA allows patients to control the amount of analgesia they receive (Ferrante, Ostheimer, and Covino, 1990). PCA can be accomplished by mouth or by the use of a special pump set to prescribed parameters to administer the drug intravenously, subcutaneously, or epidurally. In contrast to the use of PCA in postoperative pain management, the majority of the opioid dose is usually delivered via continuous systemic infusion. Patient-administered boluses are required to treat breakthrough pain and to provide a basis for more accurate and rapid upward titration of the continuous infusion rate.

Intravenous or subcutaneous PCA allows patients to accommodate transient changes in analgesic requirements (such as during dressing changes or positioning) and to tailor analgesic doses according to their own requirements. PCA is also useful in controlling pain

Table 12. Intraspinal drug delivery systems

System	Advantages	Disadvantages
Percutaneous temporary catheter	Used extensively both intraoperatively and postoperatively. Useful when prognosis is limited (< 1 month).	Mechanical problems include catheter dislodgment, kinking, or migration.
Permanent silicone-rubber epidural	Catheter implantation is a minor procedure. Dislodgment and infection less common than with temporary catheters. Can deliver bolus injections, continuous infusions, or PCA (with or without continuous delivery).	
Subcutaneous implanted injection port	Increased stability, less risk of dislodgment. Can deliver bolus injections or continuous infusions (with or without PCA).	Implantation more invasive than external catheters. Approved only for epidural catheter in U.S. Potential for infection increases with frequent injections.
Subcutaneous reservoir	Potentially, reduced infection in comparison to external system.	Difficult to access, and fibrosis may occur after repeated injection.
Implanted pumps (continuous and programmable)	Potentially, decreased risk of infection.	Need for more extensive operative procedure. Need for specialized, costly equipment with programmable systems.

quickly in the patient admitted to the hospital specifically for analgesia, and in determining the opioid dosage requirements for conversion to an oral regimen once a steady level of satisfactory analgesia is attained (Baumann, Batenhorst, Graves, et al., 1986). Intravenous and subcutaneous PCA is safe for both home and hospitalized patients (Baumann, Batenhorst, Graves, et al., 1986; Citron, Johnston-Early, Boyer, et al., 1986; Kerr, Sone, Deangelis, et al., 1988; Swanson, Smith, Bulich, et al., 1989) but is contraindicated for sedated and confused patients (Ferrell, Cronin Nash, and Warfield, 1992).

Management of Side Effects_____

Constipation and sedation are the most common side effects associated with opioids; others include confusion, nausea and vomiting, respiratory depression, dry mouth, urinary retention, pruritus, myoclonus, altered cognitive function, dysphoria, euphoria, sleep disturbances, sexual dysfunction, physiologic dependence, tolerance, and inappropriate secretion of antidiuretic hormone (Table 13). **Because there is great individual variation in the development of opioid-induced side effects, clinicians should monitor for them and prophylactically treat some inevitable ones.**

Constipation. Constipation is a common problem associated with opioid administration. Tolerance to the constipating effects of opioids either does not occur or occurs very slowly during chronic therapy. Constipation may worsen with time because of the disease process (e.g., intestinal obstruction, paralytic ileus due to spinal cord compression, decreased food and fluid intake due to anorexia); therefore a careful search for other causes should be performed (Glare and Lickiss, 1992). Mild constipation can usually be managed by an increase in fiber consumption and the use of a mild laxative such as milk of magnesia. These cathartic agents should be administered on a regular schedule, barring contraindications. Severe constipation occurs as a result of the inhibition of peristalsis by opioids and can be treated with a stimulating cathartic drug, e.g., bisacodyl, standardized senna concentrate, or hyperosmotic agents (e.g., lactulose or sorbitol). Oral laxatives can be taken at bedtime, and rectal suppositories can be used in the morning if needed.

Stool softeners or emollient laxatives, e.g., docusate, are of limited usefulness because of colonic resorption of water from the forming stool. They should not be used as the sole regimen but may be useful when given in combination with stimulant laxatives to ease defecation, especially in bedridden patients (Levy, 1991).

Sedation. Transitory sedation is common when opioid doses are increased substantially, but tolerance usually develops rapidly. Persistent drug-induced sedation is usually best treated by reducing the opioid in each dose and increasing the dosage frequency. This strategy will decrease the peak concentrations in blood (and brain) while maintaining the same total dose. In some patients, switching to another opioid may reduce the sedative effects. CNS stimulants such as caffeine, dextroamphetamine (2.5 to 7.5 mg twice daily, orally), pemoline (18.5 to 37 mg, orally), or methylphenidate (5 to 10 mg, orally) (Bruera, Brenneis, and Paterson, 1989) may be added to increase alertness if the above approach is ineffective in reducing sedation (Forrest, Brown, Brown, et al., 1977).

Table 13. General comments and cautions regarding the use of opioid analgesics

- Drugs of choice for severe cancer-related pain. Opioids do not have an analgesic ceiling effect, and therefore, dose can be titrated to achieve maximum pain relief.

- Constipation is an almost universal complication of opioid use, so all patients should receive prophylactic stimulant laxative therapy unless otherwise contraindicated (e.g., chronic diarrhea).

- Sedation is a frequent side effect of initial opioid use; however, tolerance develops soon in most patients.

- Respiratory depression rarely occurs except in opioid-naive patients and those with significant pulmonary disease.

- True hypersensitivity reactions to opioids are rare. If patients experience such reactions, it is often possible to administer an opioid from another subclass safely.

  The subclasses are: Phenanthrene derivatives: morphine, codeine, hydromorphone, oxycodone. Phenylpiperidine derivatives: meperidine, fentanyl. Diphenylheptane derivatives: methadone.

- The use of opioid antagonists such as naloxone can immediately reverse all opioid effects including analgesia. Such reversal results in acute withdrawal, which may be complicated by excruciating pain and seizure. Therefore, opioid antagonists are never recommended to reverse non-life-threatening effects such as confusion or sedation. If used to reverse life-threatening respiratory depression or hypotension, they should be titrated cautiously.

- Oral is the preferred route of administration, except for patients who cannot take or tolerate oral medications. When given in appropriate doses, oral opioids are as efficacious as parenteral opioids.

- Rectal and transdermal dosage forms are available and effective noninvasive alternatives when oral medication is not possible.

  Rectal suppositories are contraindicated if lesions of the rectum or anus are present.

- Repetitive intramuscular and subcutaneous (SC) injections should be avoided because they are painful and absorption is inconsistent.

- Intravenous (IV) administration may be used when less invasive routes are ineffective or unavailable. IV opioids may be given by bolus or continuous administration (including PCA); however, they require careful monitoring during titration. Inappropriately excessive dosing may carry significant risk of respiratory depression, especially in opioid-naive patients or those with underlying pulmonary pathology.

  Low-volume continuous SC infusion may also be used if venous access is not established.

- IV or SC PCA provides a good steady level of analgesia. It is widely accepted by patients but requires special infusion pumps and staff education. May not be appropriate for patients with altered mental status or agitation.

- Epidural and intrathecal opioids provide good analgesia, when suitable. These routes have significant risk of respiratory depression, which may be delayed, necessitating careful monitoring. Special preservative-free drug formulations are necessary for these routes of administration.

These agents also improve the cognitive function of patients receiving opioids, most likely by counteracting the sedation. In these patients, methylphenidate has been demonstrated to improve functioning on a number of neuropsychological tests, including tests of memory, mental speed, and concentration (Bruera, Miller, Macmillan, et al., 1992).

Nausea and Vomiting. There are no controlled studies that establish the indications, efficacy, and dosing requirements for treatment of opioid-induced nausea and vomiting. As with other side effects, it is important to determine the cause. Clinical experience suggests that opioid-induced nausea and vomiting can be managed with antiemetics chosen according to their modes of action. Metoclopramide is helpful when neuroleptics such as prochlorperazine, chlorpromazine, or haloperidol fail to control nausea and vomiting. Scopolamine or hydroxyzine may ameliorate symptoms as a result of their effects on the vestibular system. Scopolamine, which is an acetylcholine receptor antagonist, can be given transdermally to reduce nausea due to motion sickness (Ferris, Kerr, Sone, et al., 1991) or related to cancer. When patients complain of nausea after opioid administration has begun, it is often helpful to administer an antiemetic on a fixed schedule for several days, after which as-needed dosing is usually adequate (Portenoy, 1988). Depending on the antiemetic chosen, patients should be monitored for the possibility of increased sedation.

Respiratory Depression. Patients receiving long-term opioid therapy usually develop tolerance to the respiratory-depressant effects of these agents. Occasionally, respiratory depression occurs when pain is abruptly relieved and the sedative effects of opioids are no longer opposed by the stimulating effects of pain (Hanks, Twycross, and Lloyd, 1981). In a symptomatic patient, physical stimulation may be enough to prevent significant hypoventilation. Opioid antagonists (e.g., naloxone) should be given cautiously to patients who are receiving opioids on a long-term basis. Because patients who have become tolerant to opioids show great sensitivity to the effects of antagonist drugs, symptomatic respiratory depression should be treated carefully using a dilute solution of naloxone (0.4 mg in 10 mL of saline), administered as 0.5 mL (0.02 mg) boluses every minute. The dose of naloxone should be titrated to the patient's respiratory rate. A return to full alertness is often accompanied by a severe withdrawal syndrome and a return of pain. **Naloxone titration, when indicated for the reversal of opioid-induced respiratory depression, should be given incrementally in doses that improve respiratory function but do not reverse analgesia.** Repeated doses may be required (American Pain Society, 1992; Portenoy, 1988), or alternatively, an infusion of two ampules (total, 0.8 mg) in 250 mL of 5 percent dextrose in water may be continuously titrated toward this goal.

Far more common than acute respiratory depression is subacute overdose, in which sedation gradually builds and is followed by a slowing of respiratory rate and then by ventilatory failure. The degree of sedation rather than the respiratory rate is a better indicator of impending respiratory depression (Kaiko, Kanner, Foley, et al., 1987). The risk of this complication is highest during titration of opioids with long plasma half-lives, such as methadone and levorphanol, and is best managed by withholding one or two doses and then reducing the standing dose by 25 percent of its current level until symptoms have resolved. At that time, a cautious titration can be resumed. The maintenance of 25 percent of the dose has been found to be adequate to prevent acute opioid withdrawal (American Pain Society, 1992).

Clinicians are often concerned that high doses of opioids used for palliation may harm or kill a patient, particularly when doses are further increased to alleviate pain (Cain and Hammes, in press). This double effect of intended benefit and potential harm (Reich, 1992) is seen in the clinical situation when the intended treatment may have inextricably linked deleterious side effects. The administration of medication is always a risk-versus-benefit calculation. When the patient's death is imminent because of the progression of primary disease, an increased risk of earlier death counts little against the benefit of pain relief and painless death. The ethical duty to benefit the patient through relieving pain is by itself adequate to support increasing doses to alleviate pain, even if there might be life-shortening and expected side effects. Because many patients in the terminal phase have been receiving opioid pain medications for a significant period of time, the fear of shortening life by medication is usually unfounded. Respiratory depression is not often a significant limiting factor in pain management because, with repeated doses, tolerance develops to this effect, allowing for adequate pain treatment with escalating doses without respiratory compromise (Foley, 1991). The person dying from cancer should not be allowed to live out life with unrelieved pain because of fear of side effects; rather, appropriate, aggressive palliative support should be given (see Shapiro, in press, b; Cain and Hammes, in press).

Other Side Effects. Opioids occasionally cause myoclonus, seizures, hallucinations (Bruera, Schoeller, and Montejo, 1992), confusion, sexual dysfunction, sleep disturbances, and pruritus (Thangathurai, Bowles, Allen, et al., 1988). Prolonged use is known to affect sexual function and libido in both men and women. Women experience amenorrhea and infertility, whereas men report an inability to attain or maintain an erection. Changes in serum testosterone and other sex hormones have been described and may be responsible for some of these effects (Abel, 1984).

Urinary retention may also occur, especially with spinal opioids (Cousins and Mather, 1984; Dray, 1988; Moulin, Kreeft, Murray-Parsons, et al., 1991; Rawal, Möllefors, Axelsson, et al., 1983), in men with prostatism, or in patients with pelvic tumors and bladder outlet obstruction. The management of urinary retention may include discontinuing adjuvant drugs with potentiating effects (e.g., tricyclic antidepressants) or changing to another opioid analgesic or route of administration. Diphenhydramine, an antihistamine, may reduce pruritus in some patients. The syndrome of the inappropriate secretion of antidiuretic hormone is a rare, often transitory, adverse effect of opioid drugs, most commonly reported with morphine and methadone; more often, it is a paraneoplastic complication.

Adjuvant Drugs

Adjuvant drugs are used to enhance the analgesic efficacy of opioids, treat concurrent symptoms that exacerbate pain, and provide independent analgesia for specific types of pain. They may be used in all stages of the analgesic ladder. Commonly used agents are described below, with approximate daily dosage ranges listed in Table 14.

Corticosteroids

Corticosteroids provide a range of effects including mood elevation, anti-inflammatory activity, antiemetic activity, and appetite stimulation. These effects may be beneficial in the management of cachexia and anorexia in terminal illness (Bruera, Roca, Cedaro, et al., 1985). They also reduce cerebral and spinal cord edema and are essential in the emergency management of elevated intracranial pressure and epidural spinal cord compression. Steroids are part of the standard therapy for tumor-induced spinal cord compression (Byrne, 1992), and they are effective in reducing pain due to perineural edema and pressure on nerves. Dexamethasone (16 to 24 mg/day) or prednisone (40 to 100 mg/day) may be added to opioids for the management of pain in brachial or lumbosacral plexopathy. Undesirable effects such as myopathy, hyperglycemia, weight gain, and dysphoria may occur during prolonged steroid therapy.

Anticonvulsants

Anticonvulsants are used to manage neuropathic pain, especially when the pain is lancinating or burning. Phenytoin, carbamazepine, valproate, and clonazepam suppress spontaneous neuronal firing and are used to control lancinating pain complicating nerve injury (Swerdlow, 1984). Dose-related transient bone marrow suppression, which is associated with carbamazepine therapy (Horowitz, Patwardhan, and

Table 14. Adjuvant analgesic drugs for cancer pain

Drug	Approximate adult daily dose range	Route of administration[1]	Type of pain
Corticosteroids			
Dexamethasone[2]	16-96 mg	PO, IV	Pain associated with brain metastases and epidural spinal cord compression
Prednisone	40-100 mg	PO	
Anticonvulsants			
Carbamazepine[3]	200-1,600 mg	PO	Neuropathic pain
Phenytoin[4]	300-500 mg	PO	
Antidepressants			
Amitriptyline[5]	25-15 mg	PO	Neuropathic pain
Doxepin[6]	25-150 mg	PO	
Imipramine[7]	20-100 mg	PO	
Trazodone[8]	75-225 mg	PO	
Neuroleptics			
Methotrimeprazine[9]	40-80 mg	IM	Analgesia; sedation; antiemetic
Antihistamines			
Hydroxyzine[10]	300-450 mg	IM	Adjuvant to opioids in post-operative and other types of pain; relief of complicating symptoms including anxiety, insomnia, nausea
Local anesthestics/antiarrythmics			
Lidocaine[11]	5 mg/kg	IV/SC	Neuropathic pain
Mexiletine[12]	450-600 mg	PO	
Tocainide[13]	20 mg/kg	PO	
Psychostimulants			
Dextroamphetamine[14]	5-10 mg	PO	Improve opioid analgesia, decrease sedation
Methylphenidate[15]	10-15 mg	PO	

[1]PO=orally. IV=intravenously. IM=intramuscularly. SC=subcutaneously.
[2]French and Galicich, 1964; Greenberg, Kim, and Posner, 1980; Weissman, 1988.
[3]Lindstrom and Lindblom, 1987.
[4]Yajnik, Singh, Singh, et al., 1992.
[5]Max, Culnane, Schafer, et al., 1987; Max, Schafer, Culnane, et al., 1988; Onghena and

Marcus, 1988; Pellock, 1987), requires that it be used with caution in cancer patients undergoing other marrow-suppressant therapies, such as chemotherapy and radiation therapy. Toxicity often correlates with high concentrations in serum, and levels in serum of phenytoin, valproate, and carbamazepine should be monitored routinely (for example, monthly in the stable patient). Systemically administered local anesthetic (intravenous lidocaine, oral mexilitine, and tocainide) and antiarrhythmic agents have been used clinically to treat neuropathic pain (Brose and Cousins, 1991; Dejgard, Petersen, and Kastrup, 1988), although this is not currently an FDA-approved indication for these drugs.

Antidepressants

Tricyclic antidepressants are useful as adjuvant analgesics in the pharmacologic management of cancer pain, especially neuropathic pain. These drugs potentiate the analgesic effects of opioids in animal models of pain (Botney and Fields, 1983; Spiegel, Kalb, and Pasternak, 1983) and have innate analgesic properties (Kishore-Kumar, Max, Schafer, et al., 1990; Max, Culnane, Schafer, et al., 1987). They are effective through mechanisms that include: (1) mood elevation (France, 1987), (2) potentiation or enhancement of opioid analgesia (Ventafridda, Bianchi, Ripamonti, et al., 1990), and (3) direct analgesic effects (Max, Schafer, Culnane, et al., 1988).

The most widely reported experience has been with amitriptyline; therefore, it should be viewed as the tricyclic agent of choice, even though it produces anticholinergic side effects such as dry mouth, constipation, and urinary retention in many patients. Analgesic treatment failure may be due to low levels in serum (Max, Culnane, Schafer, et al., 1987; Max, Schafer, Culnane, et al., 1988). Doses of amitriptyline of up to 150 mg daily or higher may be required to obtain therapeutic effects (Kvinesdsal, Molin, Froland, et al., 1984; Watson

---

Van Houdenhove, 1992; Turkington, 1980; Ventafridda, Bonezzi, Caraceni, et al., 1987; Watson and Evans, 1985; Watson, Evans, Reed, et al., 1982; Young and Clarke, 1985.
[6]Cohn, Machado, Bier, et al., 1988.
[7]Kvinesdal, Molin, Froland, et al., 1984; Turkington, 1980; Young and Clarke, 1985.
[8]Khurana, 1983; Ventafridda, Bonezzi, Caraceni, et al., 1987.
[9]Beaver, Wallenstein, Houde, et al., 1966; Rogers, 1989.
[10]Beaver and Feise, 1976; Bellville, Dorey, Capparell, et al., 1979; Glazier, 1990.
[11]Bach, Jensen, Kastrup, et al., 1990; Cousins and Brose, 1991.
[12]Dejgard, Petersen, and Kastrup, 1989.
[13]Lindstrom and Lindblom, 1987.
[14]Joshi, deJongh, Schnapper, et al., 1982.
[15]Bruera, Chadwick, Brenneis, et al., 1987.

and Evans, 1985). In the treatment of diabetic neuropathy pain, the therapeutic analgesic effects of amitriptyline appear to be correlated with concentrations in serum above 100 ng/mL. However, a corresponding relationship between amitriptyline concentrations in serum and analgesia has not been reported in cancer pain.

The onset of analgesic effects occurs within 1 to 2 weeks after the start of therapy and peaks at 4 to 6 weeks (Max, Culnane, Schafer, et al., 1987; Max, Schafer, Culnane, et al., 1988; Pilowsky, Hallett, Bassett, et al., 1982). Treatment should be initiated with a small dose of amitriptyline (10 to 25 mg at bedtime), especially in debilitated patients, and increased slowly by 10 to 25 mg every 2 to 4 days toward 150 mg. This approach takes advantage of the sedative effects of the drug and minimizes the risk of falling (especially in elderly patients) because of orthostatic hypotension. Amitriptyline is also useful when sleep disturbance complicates the presence of pain and depression, because its initial use is commonly associated with sedation.

Neuroleptic Agents

Neuroleptics,which include the major tranquilizers generally used to treat psychoses and other psychiatric disorders, have also been used as adjunctive analgesics. Methotrimeprazine is a phenothiazine that has analgesic properties. Intramuscular doses of 15 mg methotrimeprazine and 10 mg of morphine are equianalgesic (Lasagna and De Kornfeld, 1961). This phenothiazine analgesic lacks opioid-inhibitory effects on gut motility and probably produces analgesia through α-adrenergic blockade (Beaver, Wallenstein, Houde, et al., 1966). In patients who are opioid tolerant or who are experiencing dose-limiting opioid side effects, especially intractable constipation, it is an alternative analgesic approach. It also has antiemetic and anxiolytic effects.

Methotrimeprazine can produce sedation and hypotension and should be given cautiously. Although it is approved only for intramuscular administration, clinicians have experience with oral and slow intravenous infusion to manage delirium, restlessness, and agitation in patients near death. Other phenothiazines have not been demonstrated to have analgesic properties (Maltbie, Cavenar, Sullivan, et al., 1979).

Hydroxyzine

Hydroxyzine is a mild anxiolytic agent with sedating and analgesic properties that is used in treating the anxious patient with pain (Beaver and Feise, 1976). This antihistamine also has antiemetic activity.

Bisphosphonates and Calcitonin

Severe bone pain is a frequent complication of bone metastases. For example, Galasko (1972) reported that 65 percent of patients with bone metastases from breast cancer experience bone pain. Bone pain is probably caused by osteoclast-induced bone resorption by the tumor, which may also result in osteoporosis, hypercalcemia, microfractures, or pathologic fractures (Ascari, Attardo-Parrinello, and Merlini, 1989). Bisphosphonates (e.g., etidronate, pamidronate) are analogues of endogenous pyrophosphates, which inhibit bone resorption in vivo (Fleish, Russel, and Francis, 1969). Pamidronate and etidronate are currently available for the management of hypercalcemia associated with malignancy. Anecdotal reports and early clinical trials have reported relief of bone pain or decreased analgesic use after the initiation of a bisphosphonate (Delmas, Charhon, Chapuy, et al., 1982; Elomaa, Blomqvist, Grohn, et al., 1983). Other researchers have described similar findings with bisphosphonates that are not available in the United States (Attardo-Parrinello, Merlini, Pavesi, et al., 1987; van Holten-Verzantvoort, Zwinderman, Aaronson, et al., 1991). Smith (1989), however, reported no difference in symptomatic relief or analgesic requirements in 57 patients with advanced hormone-refractory prostate cancer treated with etidronate or placebo.

Calcitonin is also a potent inhibitor of osteoclast-induced bone resorption and, like the bisphosphonates, is used in the management of hypercalcemia of malignancy. At least one double-blind, randomized trial comparing salmon calcitonin to placebo demonstrated that 100 IU/day subcutaneously resulted in reduced analgesic consumption, shorter duration of pain, and subjective improvement (Roth and Kolaric, 1986).

Although these agents that inhibit bone resorption appear to be beneficial in some patients with painful bone metastases, other patients have failed to respond. Additional studies are warranted to define criteria that may predict a clinical response to these drugs and to define further their optimal use in this setting.

Placebos

A mention of the placebo response is important to highlight the potentially harmful misunderstanding surrounding this phenomenon. The placebo response is common, and placebo-derived analgesia may be mediated to a great extent through endogenous opioid pathways. The deceptive use of placebo response to distinguish psychogenic pain from "real" pain should be avoided. **Placebos are effective in a portion of patients for a short period of time only and should not be used in the management of cancer pain (American Pain Society, 1992; Foley, 1985a; World Health Organization, 1990).**

Antineoplastic Therapies

Antineoplastic treatments for cancer include chemotherapy, hormonal and biologic therapies, and radiotherapy. Chemotherapy and hormonal therapies are generally used to treat all sites of cancer throughout the body and are not used specifically to treat pain. However, when the cause of cancer pain is direct tumor involvement, antineoplastic treatments may produce analgesia if they cause significant tumor shrinkage.

The major goal of antineoplastic treatment is either to cure by complete elimination of the cancer or, in situations in which cure is not possible, to prolong life and to achieve palliation of the tumor symptoms. Most important, the patient and clinician should discuss openly and thoroughly the expected goals and potential side effects of these therapies.

Influence of Concurrent Medical Conditions on Pharmacotherapy

The presence of other medical conditions in cancer patients and the medications taken for them may influence the choice of analgesic regimen for pain management. Common medications or classes of medications that produce clinically significant drug interactions with opioid analgesics include alcohol (as in elixirs) and other CNS depressants such as phenytoin, as well as rifampin (Kreek, Garfield, Gutjahr, et al., 1976) and monoamine oxidase inhibitors such as phenylzine sulfate and isocarboxazid (Breitbart and Holland, 1988).

Coexisting conditions also may influence the type and doses of opioid analgesics administered. For example, patients with newly recognized cancer pain who have been recently treated with opioids for another reason, such as surgery, may require higher than the recommended starting doses because they are opioid tolerant. Coagulopathy, neutropenia, and sepsis may contraindicate the use of epidural catheters or other regional anesthetic techniques because the risks of bleeding or "seeding" of infection are increased.

Many patients with cancer undergo surgery as part of their treatment. GI procedures such as gastrectomy and colectomy may markedly affect drug absorption and increase GI intolerance to some oral drugs. Drug pharmacokinetics can change after surgery because of changes in drug absorption and distribution caused by alterations in body weight, cardiac output, venous capacitance, extravascular fluid shifts, and protein binding. Fever and sepsis in the postoperative period can affect drug disposition, as do shock or trauma. Patients with such conditions may require higher than expected doses of opioids because of severe acute pain. In addition, they may not achieve clinically effective concentrations of opioids in plasma after intramuscular and subcutaneous injections because of the pharmaco-kinetic alterations described above.

Cancer often occurs in the elderly, who usually have decreased renal function as a normal result of aging. Mild age-related renal insufficiency (decline in glomerular filtration rate) can impede the excretion of the biologically active metabolites of many opioids, resulting in clinically significant sedation and respiratory depression (Sear, Hand, Moore, et al., 1989), as well as nausea (Hagen, Foley, Cerbone, et al., 1991). Meperidine, methadone, levorphano, penta-zocine, and propoxyphene have increased bioavailability, prolonged half-lives, and decreased systemic clearance and thus accumulate in patients with hepatic or renal dysfunction. Renal excretion is a major route of elimination not only for opioids but also for their pharmaco-logically active metabolites norpropoxyphene, normeperidine, morphine-6-glucuronide, and dihydrocodeine. Hence, in patients with renal dysfunction, doses of the parent compounds should be lowered or given less frequently.

Pharmacologic Treatments Not Recommended

A number of drugs and routes of administration are not recom-mended for the relief of cancer pain. These are summarized in Table 15.

Discharge Planning Regarding Medications

Patients and their families may have difficulty in understanding and remembering the details of the plan for managing pain. Therefore, **patients should be given a written pain management plan** (Figure 5, see page 74). Pertinent instructions related to the management of pain include the specific drugs to be taken; the type and purpose of pain medication (e.g., opioid, tricyclic antidepressant, anxiolytic); the frequency of drug administration, with an emphasis in most cases on taking the medication around the clock rather than as needed; poten-tial side effects of each pain medication (particularly constipation for opioids) and a plan for their prevention or treatment; potential drug interactions; specific precautions to follow when taking a pain medica-tion, such as physical activity limitations and dietary restrictions; and whom to notify about pain problems or concerns about the medication.

The plan should be reviewed with the patient, and the patient and/or caregiver should be given an opportunity to discuss fears or concerns about the use of opioid analgesics; to clarify issues related to tolerance, dependence, and addiction; to voice concerns about side

Table 15. Drugs and routes of administration not recommended for treatment of cancer pain

Class	Drug	Rationale for not recommending
Opioids	Meperidine	Short (2-3 hour) duration. Repeated administration may lead to CNS toxicity (tremor, confusion, or seizures) (Cleeland, 1985; Kaiko, Foley, Grabinski, et al., 1983; Szeto, Inturrisi, Houde, et al., 1977). High oral doses required to relieve severe pain, and these increase the risk of CNS toxicity (American Pain Society, 1992; Weissman, Burchman, Dinndorf, et al., 1992).
Miscellaneous	Cannabinoids	Side effects of dysphoria, drowsiness, hypotension, and bradycardia preclude its routine use as an analgesic (American Pain Society, 1992).
	Cocaine	Has demonstrated no efficacy as an analgesic or coanalgesic in combination with opioids (American Pain Society, 1992).
Opioid agonist-antagonists	Pentazocine Butorphanol Nalbuphine	Risk of precipitating withdrawal in opioid-dependent patients. Analgesic ceiling (Kallos and Caruso, 1979; Nagashima, Karamanian, Malovany, et al., 1976). Possible production of unpleasant psychomimetic effects (e.g., dysphoria, hallucinations) (American Pain Society, 1992; Martin, 1984; Weissman, Burchman, Dinndorf, et al., 1992).
Partial agonist	Buprenorphine	Analgesic ceiling. Can precipitate withdrawal (American Pain Society, 1992; Weissman, Burchman, Dinndorf, et al., 1992).
Antagonist	Naloxone Naltrexone	May precipitate withdrawal. Limit use to treatment of life-threatening respiratory depression (Ellison, 1993).

effects; and to discuss when it is appropriate to communicate with a clinician regarding the need for a change in the plan.

Discharge planners should advise patients and clinicians to communicate the plan to other clinicians when the patient is being transferred from one health care setting to another, such as being discharged from an acute care facility to a hospice, in order to maintain continuity in pain management. Attachment B contains examples of forms that patients can use at home to document their pain.

Class	Drug	Rationale for not recommending
Combination preparations	Brompton's cocktail	No evidence of analgesic benefit to using Brompton's cocktail over single opioid analgesics (Twycross, 1977; Walsh, 1984; Weissman, Burchman, Dinndorf, et al., 1992; Wisconsin Cancer Pain Initiative, 1988).
	DPT (Meperidine, Promethazine, and Chlorpromazine)	Efficacy is poor compared with that of other analgesics. High incidence of adverse effects (Nahata, Clotz, and Krogg, 1985).
Anxiolytics alone	Benzodiazepine (e.g., alprazolam)	Analgesic properties not demonstrated except for some instances of neuropathic pain. Added sedation from anxiolytics may limit opioid dosing (American Pain Society, 1992; Weissman, Burchman, Dinndorf, et al., 1992).
Sedative/ hypnotic drugs alone	Barbiturates Benzodiazepine	Analgesic properties not demonstrated. Added sedation from sedative/hypnotic drugs limits opioid dosing (American Pain Society, 1992).

Routes of administration	Rationale for not recommending
Intramuscular (IM)	Painful. Absorption unreliable (American Pain Society, 1992). Should not be used for children or patients prone to develop dependent edema or in patients with thrombocytopenia (Weissman, Burchman, Dinndorf, et al., 1992).
Transnasal	The only drug approved by the FDA for transnasal administration at this time is butorphanol, an agonist-antagonist drug, which generally is not recommended. (See opioid agonist-antagonists above.)

Figure 5. Pain management plan

Pain control plan for

_____

At home, I will take the following medicines for pain control:

Medicine	How to take	How many	How often	Comments
_____	_____	_____	_____	_____
_____	_____	_____	_____	_____
_____	_____	_____	_____	_____
_____	_____	_____	_____	_____

Medicines that you may take to help treat side effects:

Side effect	Medicine	How to take	How many	How often	Comments
_____	_____	_____	_____	_____	_____
_____	_____	_____	_____	_____	_____

Constipation is a very common problem when taking opioid medications. When this occurs, do the following:

❑ Increase fluid intake (8 to 10 glasses of fluid)
❑ Exercise regularly
❑ Increase fiber in the diet (bran, fresh fruits, vegetables)
❑ Use a mild laxative, such as milk of magnesia, if no bowel movement in 3 days
❑ Take _____ every day at _____ (time) with a full glass of water
❑ Use a glycerin suppository every morning (this may help make a bowel movement less painful)

Non-drug pain control methods:

_____

_____

Additional instructions:

_____

_____

_____

Important phone numbers:

Your doctor_____   Your nurse_____
Your pharmacy_____   Emergencies _____

Call your doctor or nurse immediately if your pain increases or if you have a new pain. Also call your doctor early for refill of pain medicines. Do not let your medicines get below 3 or 4 days' supply.

4 Nonpharmacologic Management: Physical and Psychological Modalities

Recommendations

31. Cutaneous stimulation techniques, including applications of superficial heat and cold, massage, pressure or vibration, should be offered to alleviate pain associated with muscle tension or muscle spasm. (C)

32. Patients should be encouraged to remain active and to participate in self-care when possible. (A)

33. Clinicians should reposition patients on a scheduled basis during long-term bedrest and provide active and passive range-of-motion exercises. For a patient in acute pain, exercise should be limited to self-administered range of motion. (C)

34. Prolonged immobilization should be avoided whenever possible to prevent joint contracture, muscle atrophy, cardiovascular deconditioning, and other untoward effects. (B)

35. Patients who choose to have acupuncture for pain management should be encouraged to report new pain problems to their health care team before seeking palliation through acupuncture. (Panel Consensus)

36. Psychosocial interventions should be introduced early in the course of illness as part of a multimodal approach to pain management. They generally should not be used as substitutes for analgesics. (A)

37. Because of the many misconceptions regarding pain and its treatment, education about the ability to control pain effectively and correction of myths about the use of opioids should be included as part of the treatment plan for all patients. (B)

38. Clinicians should offer patients and families means to contact peer support groups. (Panel Consensus)

39. Pastoral care members should participate in health care team meetings that discuss the needs and treatment of patients. They should develop information about community resources that provide the spiritual care and support of patients and their families. (Panel Consensus)

Introduction

Physical and psychosocial therapies can be used concurrently with drugs and other modalities to manage pain. These interventions can be carried out by professional staff and often by the patient or family members.

Physical Modalities

Physical modalities include cutaneous stimulation, exercise, immobilization, transcutaneous electrical nerve stimulation (TENS), and acupuncture (Lee, Itoh, Yang, et al., 1990). Their use may decrease the need for pain-reducing drugs, but they should not be used as substitutes for medication. These modalities should be introduced early to treat generalized weakness and deconditioning as well as aches and pains associated with periods of inactivity and immobility related to cancer diagnosis and therapy.

Cutaneous Stimulation

Cutaneous stimulation includes the application of superficial heat (thermotherapy) and cold (cryotherapy) (Mayer, 1985). Other methods, such as massage, pressure, and vibration, may help patients to relax or distract them from their pain. Cutaneous stimulation sometimes increases pain briefly before pain relief occurs (McCaffery and Beebe, 1989). These methods are noninvasive and usually can be easily taught to the patient or family caregiver.

Superficial applications of heat act through conduction or convection to increase the blood flow to the skin and superficial organs and to decrease the blood flow to inactive tissues such as the underlying musculature (Lehmann and de Lateur, 1990). Heat induces vasodilation, which increases oxygen and nutrient delivery to damaged tissues (Whitney, 1989). Heat also decreases joint stiffness by increasing the elastic properties of muscles (Vasudevan, Hegmann, Moore, et al., 1992). Superficial heat can be applied by hot packs, hot water bottles, hot and moist compresses, electric heating pads (dry or moist), commercially available chemical and gel packs, and immersion in water (tub, basin, or whirlpool) (McCaffery and Wolff, 1992). For all types of hot packs, care should be taken to wrap them well to prevent burns and to discourage patients from lying directly on them. In most cases, the protection of one towel between the skin and the heating device is sufficient. If the patient has decreased skin sensation, is using an electrical heating device, or tends to lie on top of a hot pack, more layers of cloth are needed for skin protection and close monitoring of the skin condition is required. Heat should not be applied to tissue that has been exposed to radiation therapy.

The literature is divided on the use of heat in patients with cancer. Superficial heat is commonly used by patients to reduce pain (Barbour, McGuire, and Kirchhoff, 1986; Davis, Cortex, and Rubin, 1990; Donovan and Dillon, 1987; Rhiner, Ferrell, Ferrell, et al., 1993; Wilkie, Lovejoy, Dodd, et al., 1988), and some texts recommend heat to reduce pain and discomfort (Ferrell, Rhiner, and Ferrell, 1993; McCaffery and Wolff, 1992; Vasudevan, Hegmann, Moore, et al., 1992). Other texts, however, caution against the use of heat because of concern that the use of heat over tumor sites will increase tumor growth and the metastatic spread of the disease (Lee, Itoh, Yang, et al., 1990; Lehmann and de Lateur, 1990; Pfalzer, 1992). Research evidence cited in support of this cautionary statement is from a 1940 study of rats (Hayashi, 1940), as well as several studies of fetal tissue cells exposed to high degrees of temperature (Lehmann and de Lateur, 1990).

In view of the lack of research findings that clearly contraindicate this use of superficial heat, the panel recommends that it be used as a method of pain control in patients with cancer. Modalities to deliver deep heat—such as short wave diathermy, microwave diathermy, and ultrasound—should be used with caution in patients with active cancer; they should not be applied directly over a cancer site (Lehmann and de Lateur, 1990).

Cold therapy, which causes vasoconstriction and local hyperesthesia, is effective in reducing inflammation, edema soon after an injury, burning perineal pain (Evans, Lloyd, and Jack, 1981), and muscle spasm (Vasudevan, Hegmann, Moore, et al., 1992), and is recommended when superficial heat is ineffective in reducing spasm. Ice packs, towels soaked in ice water, or commercially prepared chemical gel packs can be used. Cold packs should be sealed to prevent dripping, they should be flexible to conform to body contours, they should be applied so as to produce a comfortable and safe intensity of cold, and they should be adequately wrapped (e.g., in one layer of towel or pillowcase) to prevent skin irritation. The duration of ice application is shorter than that of heat, usually lasting less than 15 minutes; however, it produces a longer acting effect, provided that the muscle is actually cooled (Lehmann and de Lateur, 1990; Michlovitz, 1990).

Cold should not be applied to tissue that has been damaged by radiation therapy and is contraindicated for any condition in which vasoconstriction increases symptoms, such as in peripheral vascular disease, Raynaud's syndrome, or other vascular or connective tissue diseases (Lehmann and de Lateur, 1990; Whitney, 1989). In some patients, cooling painful joints will increase range of motion, but in others, this may increase joint stiffness and should therefore be avoided.

Massage is a comfort measure used to aid relaxation and ease general aches and pains, particularly those associated with periods of treatment related immobility. Massage may also decrease pain in a specific area by increasing superficial circulation (Fairchild, Salerno, Wedding, et al., 1986; McCaffery and Wolff, 1992). Common techniques of massage are stroking, kneading, and rubbing with rhythmic, circular, distal-to-proximal motions (Lee, Itoh, Yang, et al., 1990). An alcohol-free lotion can be used to reduce friction. The patient should be encouraged to choose movements that provide the greatest comfort. Massage cannot strengthen debilitated muscles, and it should not be used in place of exercise and activity for patients who are able to walk. Manual or mechanical vibration can also be used to increase superficial circulation. Specific instructions for the use of a variety of cutaneous stimulation methods for pain relief are available elsewhere (McCaffery and Beebe, 1989). An example of a relaxation technique that uses massage, touch, and warmth is included in Attachment C.

Exercise

Exercise is important for the treatment of subacute and chronic pain because it strengthens weak muscles, mobilizes stiff joints, helps restore coordination and balance, enhances patient comfort, and provides cardiovascular conditioning (Vasudevan, Hegmann, Moore, et al., 1992). Barbour, McGuire, and Kirchhoff (1986) found that some patients use position change or exercise as a self-initiated strategy for pain relief; of those who used these strategies, 86 percent reported pain relief with change of position and 25 percent reported pain relief after exercise. **Patients should be encouraged to remain active and participate in self-care when possible** (Kohl, LaPorte and Blair, 1988; Kovar, Allegrante, MacKenzie, et al., 1992; Powell, Thompson, Caspersen, et al., 1987; Siscovick, LaPorte, and Newman, 1985).

When patients are unable to maintain function, families should be taught a simple routine of range-of-motion exercises and massage to minimize discomfort and preserve muscle length and joint function during periods of decreased function and immobility (Kisner and Colby, 1985). Passive exercises should not be carried out if they increase pain. **During acute pain, exercise should be limited to self-administered range of motion** (Lee, Itoh, Yang, et al., 1990). All forms of exercise that involve weight bearing should be avoided when pathologic fracture is likely because of tumor invasion.

Positioning is another simple method to promote comfort and to prevent or relieve pain. Clinicians should ensure that patients who are bedridden are positioned in correct body alignment, that patients are repositioned frequently, that skin condition is monitored, and that range-of-motion exercises are provided. Clinicians should educate ancillary personnel and family caregivers so that they are able to perform range of motion exercises correctly and safely position patients.

Immobilization or restriction of movement is often used to manage episodes of acute pain and to stabilize fractures or otherwise compromised limbs, joints, or both. When immobility is desired, supportive devices such as adjustable elastic or thermoplastic braces can be used to maintain optimal body alignment. Joints should not be maintained at their maximal range but in their position of optimal function (i.e., wrist at 30° of dorsiflexion with thumb opposed to fingers, ankle at 90° flexion with 5° to 10° flexion of the knee, etc.) to allow for maximal function after an immobilization period (Lee, Itoh, Yang, et al., 1990). In patients with bone metastasis, immobilization may be necessary to prevent fractures. These patients and their families should be taught how to apply orthotic devices properly and how to prevent torsion during positioning and turning. **Prolonged immobilization should be avoided whenever possible to prevent joint contracture, muscle atrophy, cardiovascular deconditioning, and other untoward effects.**

Counterstimulation

Counterstimulation denotes techniques, such as TENS therapy and acupuncture, that are believed to activate endogenous pain-modulating pathways by direct stimulation of peripheral nerves (Sjölund and Eriksson, 1979). The literature in support of these interventions is inconclusive, although some patients report that they obtain relief from their use (Avellanosa and West, 1982; Bauer, 1983).

Transcutaneous Electrical Nerve Stimulation (TENS). TENS is a method of applying controlled, low-voltage electrical stimulation to large, myelinated peripheral nerve fibers via cutaneous electrodes for the purpose of modulating stimulus transmission and relieving pain. Research on TENS therapy in patients with cancer is limited to single-group studies and case reports (Avellanosa and West, 1982; Bauer, 1983). A meta-analysis of studies of TENS therapy in postoperative patients (Acute Pain Management Guideline Panel, in press) found that both TENS and sham TENS significantly reduced pain intensity; no significant differences were found between the two for either analgesic use or pain intensity. These results suggest that, just as with some other interventions, part of the efficacy of TENS can be attributed to a placebo effect. Patients with mild pain may benefit from a trial of TENS.

Acupuncture. Acupuncture is a neurostimulatory technique that treats pain by the insertion of small, solid needles into the skin at varying depths, typically penetrating the underlying musculature. There are few controlled studies of its use; recent meta-analyses (Patel, Gutzwiller, Paccaud, et al., 1989; ter Riet, Kleijnen, and

Knipschild, 1990) are inconclusive and do not specify which types of pain problems acupuncture can or cannot alleviate.

Pain can signal disease progression, the emergence of adventitious infection, or some significant complication of treatment. Therefore, **patients who choose to have acupuncture for pain management should be encouraged to report new pain problems to their health care team before seeking palliation through acupuncture.** Maintaining an open and accepting relationship will make it easier for the patient and the practitioner to discuss negative as well as positive experiences and situations where acupuncture might be contraindicated.

When a patient seeks TENS therapy or acupuncture, clinicians should listen for clues that would indicate that the pain is uncontrolled. If the patient is seeking these modalities because of poorly managed pain, the clinician, in cooperation with the patient, should revise the pain management plan by:

- Correcting misconceptions the patient might have concerning the use of analgesic drugs, especially the phenomena of addiction and tolerance with opioids.

- Increasing an analgesic dosage.

- Adding an adjuvant drug to manage a specific pain complaint or to counteract a side effect.

- Prescribing a psychotropic drug to manage coexisting anxiety or depression.

- Providing training in the use of cognitive-behavioral strategies.

Controlled studies are needed to test the effectiveness of counterstimulation in the treatment of cancer-related pain.

Psychosocial Interventions

Psychosocial interventions are an important part of a multimodal approach to pain management. Such interventions do not replace, but rather, are used in conjunction with appropriate analgesics for the management of pain. When psychosocial interventions are successful in relieving pain, clinicians should never conclude that the pain was not "real."

One goal is to help the patient gain a sense of control over the pain. A simple rationale underlies such intervention: How people think affects how they feel, and changing how they think about pain can change their sensitivity to it and their feelings and reactions toward it (McGrath, 1990b).

Psychosocial intervention may use cognitive or behavioral techniques or both. Focusing on perception and thought, cognitive techniques are designed to influence how one interprets events and bodily sensations. Giving patients information about pain and its management and helping patients to think differently about their pain are both cognitive techniques. Behavioral techniques, by contrast, are directed at helping patients develop skills to cope with pain and helping them modify their reactions to pain.

Many patients with cancer are highly motivated to use cognitive-behavioral methods, which are often effective not only in controlling symptoms, but also in restoring the patient's sense of self-control, personal efficacy, and active participation in his/her own care.

In recommending psychosocial interventions, the clinician should consider:

■ Intensity of pain.

■ Expected duration of pain.

■ Patient's mental clarity.

■ Patient's past experience with the technique.

■ Patient's physical ability.

■ Patient's desire to employ active or passive techniques.

Psychosocial interventions should be introduced early in the course of illness so that patients can learn and practice these strategies while they have sufficient strength and energy. When introduced early, they are more likely to succeed, which fosters the patient's motivation to continue using them. Patients and their families should be given information that describes strategies commonly used to manage pain and anxiety and encouraged to try several strategies, then select one or more to use regularly when they experience pain.

As with other modalities, psychosocial interventions can require different levels of training and expertise on the part of clinicians. The interventions discussed here, however, can be performed by most clinicians. In addition to these interventions, some patients will benefit from short-term psychotherapy (see Chapter 7).

Relaxation and Imagery

Relaxation techniques and imagery are used to achieve a state of mental and physical relaxation. Mental relaxation means alleviation of anxiety; physical relaxation means reduction in skeletal muscle tension. Relaxation techniques include simple focused-breathing exercises, progressive muscle relaxation, meditation, and music-assisted relaxation (McCaffery and Beebe, 1989) (Attachment C). Simple relaxation techniques should be used for episodes of brief pain, e.g., during procedures, as well as when the patient's ability to concentrate is compromised by severe pain, a high level of anxiety, or fatigue.

Pleasant mental images can be used to aid relaxation. For example, patients might be encouraged to visualize a peaceful scene, such as waves softly hitting the beach, or to take slow, deep breaths as they visualize pain leaving the body. Both pleasant imagery and progressive muscle relaxation have been shown to decrease self-reported pain intensity and pain distress (Graffam and Johnson, 1987).

Relaxation techniques are most helpful when combined with imagery, especially when the image is individualized to the patient's needs or preferences (Syrjala, in press). The advantages include:

- They are easy to learn.

- No special equipment is required.

- Staff do not require extensive training.

- They are often readily accepted by patients (Hendler and Redd, 1986; Syrjala, 1990).

Tapes and other resources are available for teaching relaxation (McCaffery and Beebe, 1989; Syrjala, 1990).

Distraction and Reframing

Distraction is the strategy of focusing one's attention on stimuli other than pain or the accompanying negative emotions (McCaffery and Beebe, 1989; McCaul and Malott, 1984). Distractions may be internal, for example, counting, singing mentally to one's self, praying, or making self-statements such as "I can cope," or external, for example, listening to music as an aid to relaxation (Beck, 1991; Munro and Mount, 1978), watching television, talking to family and friends, or listening to someone read. Distraction exercises often include repetitive actions or cognitive activity, such as rhythmic massage or the use of a visual focal point. Distraction may be used alone to manage mild pain or as an adjunct to analgesic drugs to manage brief episodes of severe pain, such as procedure-related pain.

A related technique, reframing or cognitive reappraisal, teaches patients to monitor and evaluate negative thoughts and images and replace them with more positive ones. For example, patients who are preoccupied with a fear of pain can be encouraged to use positive self-statements to facilitate coping (e.g., "I've had similar pain and it's gotten better"). Reframing can add to patients' feelings of control over their situations (see Attachment C).

Patient Education_____

Patient education entails giving patients and families accurate and understandable information about pain, pain assessment, and the use of drugs and other methods of pain relief, emphasizing that almost all pain can be effectively managed. It should also address major barriers to effective pain management, namely, patients' reluctance to talk about their pain with their care providers, their unfounded fears about becoming addicted to opioids, and their fears that the pain cannot be effectively controlled without unacceptable consequences. Patient education should address other misconceptions, such as the thought that pain medication should be saved for when pain is severe, or else it might not be effective (Ward, Goldberg, Miller-McCauley, et al., 1993). Some believe that analgesics might produce unacceptable side effects or that choices might have to be made between treating the disease or treating the pain.

A goal of patient education is to involve patients in their pain management: one of the most important steps toward improved control of cancer pain is better understanding by patients of the nature of the pain, its treatment, and the role that they need to play in pain control. Patients should be encouraged to report pain as active participants in their own care. To improve their understanding of drug therapy and its effects, patients should be told that:

- The use of opioid analgesics will not lead to addiction.

- Tolerance to opioid analgesics can be dealt with by upward dosage adjustments.

Many patients worry that, if they complain of pain, their health care providers might not think of them as "good" patients (Ward, Goldberg, Miller-McCauley, et al., 1993). Because of these concerns, some patients who are taking opioids and have been told to take them regularly may take them only when their pain is severe. Patients should be taught that the prevention of pain by the use of regularly scheduled analgesics is desirable. **Because of the many misconceptions regarding pain and its treatment, education about the ability to control pain effectively and correction of myths about the use of opioids should be included as part of the treatment plan.**

Table 16 specifies some of the major topics of a patient education program. The literature indicates that, to have the desired effect, information should be presented more than once and, because patients seek information from multiple sources, in more than one way.

Because uncertainty increases distress and threatens the perception of ability to cope, informing patients about what is going to happen to them can help them think about a situation differently and

Table 16. Patient education program content

General overview

Pain can be relieved.

Defining pain.

Understanding the causes of pain.

Pain assessment and use of pain-rating scales to communicate pain.

Talking to doctors and nurses about pain.

Using a preventive approach to pain control.

Pharmacologic management

Overview of drug management of pain.

Overcoming fears of addiction and drug tolerance.

Understanding drug tolerance.

Understanding respiratory depression.

Controlling common side effects of drugs (e.g., nausea and constipation).

Nonpharmacologic management

Importance of nonpharmacologic interventions.

Use of nonpharmacologic modalities as adjuncts to analgesics.

Review of previous experience with nonpharmacologic modalities.

Peer support groups and pastoral counseling.

Demonstration of heat, cold, massage, relaxation, imagery, and distraction.

Source: Ferrell, Rhiner, and Ferrell, 1993.

feel less helpless (Mishel, 1984). Research has shown that patients who receive medication-related education have a higher rate of compliance with analgesic prescriptions, fewer concerns about taking opioid analgesics, and lower pain levels than do patients not given such information (Rimer, Levy, Keintz, et al., 1987). Other research has demonstrated that informing patients about possible side effects of therapy will not increase the occurrence of side effects or have other adverse effects (Howland, Baker, and Poe, 1990; Wilson, 1981).

After the clinician has told patients that they are expected to take an active role in their pain management and has reassured them that pain relief is an important goal, then patients should be able to use clinicians as sources of information and reassurance about pain control. Information presented orally to patients should be supplemented with written material (Table 17). Additional information is included in a discussion of discharge planning in Chapter 3.

Table 17. Sources of information for patients and their families

Cancer Pain Can Be Relieved.
Wisconsin Cancer Pain Initiative; 1988, p. 10.[1]

This booklet gives clear and concise answers to 21 questions frequently asked by people with cancer pain. Topics include communicating pain to health providers, analgesics available to relieve pain, and management of side effects associated with opioid analgesics.

Children's Cancer Pain Can Be Relieved.
Wisconsin Cancer Pain Initiative; 1989, p. 12.[1]

This booklet is written for parents of children who have cancer and discusses many issues that confront children in pain and their families. A question-and-answer format is used to explain the assessment of pain in infants and children, the use of analgesics, and the management of side effects. Resources for families of children with cancer also are included.

Jeff Asks About Cancer Pain.
Wisconsin Cancer Pain Initiative; 1990, p. 12.[1]

This booklet addresses accurately and candidly the needs of adolescents who have cancer pain. It includes myths regarding addiction, methods for relieving side effects of opioids, and instructions for taking opioid analgesics during school hours. Adolescents will appreciate the language and style.

Questions and Answers About Pain Control: A Guide for People With Cancer and Their Families. American Cancer Society and the National Cancer Institute; 1992, p. 76.[2]

This book provides in-depth and current information in an easy-to-understand, question-and-answer format. Information is included on pain assessment, nonprescription and prescription medications, and nondrug interventions such as relaxation, imagery, and applications of superficial heat and cold. Common fears related to opioid analgesics (i.e., safety, addiction) are discussed, and tips for managing side effects of opioid analgesics are provided.

Facing Forward: A Guide for Cancer Survivors.
U.S. Department of Health and Human Services, Public Health Service, National Institutes of Health, National Cancer Institute, July 1990. NIH Publication No. 90-2424, p. 43.[2]

This booklet was developed to give cancer survivors practical ideas to help cope with common concerns. The topics covered are: continuing to care for your health; taking care of your feelings; managing insurance issues; and earning a living. Experiences of other cancer survivors are included, as well as facts, practical tips, options for taking control of your situation, and other resources that may be useful.

Teamwork: The Cancer Patient's Guide to Talking With Your Doctor. National Coalition for Cancer Survivorship, 1991, p. 32.[3]

This booklet is written by cancer survivors and doctors to help other patients with cancer learn how to communicate effectively with their doctors. Topics include what to tell your doctor about yourself; what doctors wish their patients knew; understanding (and remembering!) what the doctor says; and key questions to ask your doctor throughout the process, from before the diagnosis through all stages of treatment.

---

[1] Available from the Wisconsin Cancer Pain Initiative, 3675 Medical Sciences Center, 1300 University Avenue, Madison, WI 53706. Phone: (608) 262-0978.
[2] Available from local units and chapters of the American Cancer Society, Phone: 1-800-ACS-2345. Also available from the National Cancer Institute. Phone: 1-800-4-CANCER.
[3] Available from the National Coalition for Cancer Survivorship, 1010 Wayne Avenue, 5th Floor, Silver Spring, MD 20910. Phone: (301) 650-8868.
Source: Adapted with permission from Paice, 1990.

Psychotherapy and Structured Support

Some patients benefit from short-term psychotherapy or more complex cognitive-behavioral interventions provided by a psychiatrist, clinical psychologist, psychiatric nurse, or psychiatric social worker. Short-term supportive psychotherapy based on a crisis intervention model can provide emotional support, continuity, and information while helping the patient adapt to the crisis. The therapist emphasizes the patient's past strengths, supports the patient's use of previously successful coping strategies, and teaches new coping skills. Studies have shown that patients with cancer who receive active, structured psychological support report less pain and live longer (Fawzy, Cousins, Fawzy, et al., 1990; Spiegel and Bloom, 1983; Spiegel, Bloom, Kraemer, et al., 1989). Psychotherapy should be offered to patients whose pain is particularly difficult to manage (e.g., substance abusers), those who develop symptoms of clinical depression or another adjustment disorder, and those with a history of psychiatric illness.

Hypnosis

The hypnotic trance is a state of heightened awareness and focused concentration that can be used to manipulate the perception of pain and has been effective in the treatment of cancer-related pain (Reeves, Redd, Storm, et al., 1983; Spiegel and Bloom, 1983; Syrjala, Cummings, and Donaldson, 1992). It should only be administered by specially trained professionals.

Peer Support Groups

Programs of self-help and mutual support of patients with cancer have been available since the 1940s, when the American Cancer Society (ACS) established visitor programs to offer practical help for patients at home (Mastrovito, Moynihan, and Parsonnet, 1989). Some, such as the National Coalition for Cancer Survivorship and many of their local chapters, enroll survivors of any type of cancer and their relatives. Others target specific cancers; these include the International Association of Laryngectomees, the United Ostomy Association, and the ACS's Reach to Recovery program for breast surgery patients. Many of the peer support groups work closely with health care teams who refer patients to them.

The experience and empathy of people who have experienced a disease can provide credible support to others with the same disease or problem and can help new patients learn to cope more effectively (Mantell, Alexander, and Kleiman, 1976). Support networks can also help patients to maintain social identity and provide emotional

Table 18. How to find local support groups

Call the local unit of the American Cancer Society; see the phone book in the business white pages.

Contact the National Coalition for Cancer Survivorship:
  1010 Wayne Avenue, 5th Floor
  Silver Spring, MD 20910
  (301) 650-8868

Call the National Cancer Information Service, 1-800-4-CANCER.

Call the State self-help clearinghouse; the American Self-Help Clearinghouse at (201)642-7101 has information on State clearinghouses.

Contact the social service department of cancer treatment centers, an oncology social worker, or cancer counselor.

Call the local mental health department.

Check local newspapers for weekly listings.

Call the local United Way office or other community fund offices.

---

support, material aid, and access to information (Walker, MacBride, and Vachon, 1977). **Because of the benefits provided by these groups, clinicians should know which are active in their area and provide this information to patients who wish to join them.** Table18 provides suggestions on how to find a support group.

Pastoral Counseling

Having cancer and pain frequently raises issues of spirituality for patients and their families, both of whom may be helped by pastoral counseling. The experience of pain can often lead patients to fear abandonment and to question meaning and the possibility of hope. Many religions address these concerns and offer an important dimension in a multidisciplinary approach to pain management. Thus:

- **Ecumenical pastoral care should be made available.**

- **Pastoral care members should participate in health care team meetings that discuss the needs and treatment of patients.**

- **Pastoral care members should develop information about community resources that provide spiritual care and support.**

5 Nonpharmacologic Interventions: Invasive Therapies

Recommendations

40. With rare exception, noninvasive treatments should precede invasive palliative approaches. (Panel Consensus)

41. Indications for palliative radiation therapy include treatment of symptomatic metastases in sites where tumor infiltration has caused pain, obstruction, bleeding, or compression. (B)

42. Radiopharmaceuticals emitting a β-particle should be used for the pain of bone metastases only when bone scintigraphy shows a lesion. (A)

43. Radiation tolerance of adjacent normal tissues should be considered in the design of treatment portals and the prescription of teletherapy or radiopharmaceutical dose. (A)

44. The desired dosage of radiation should be administered in the fewest fractions possible to promote patient comfort during and after treatment. (Panel Consensus)

45. Neurolytic blockade of peripheral nerves should be reserved with rare exception for instances in which other therapies (palliative radiation, TENS, pharmacotherapy) are ineffective, poorly tolerated, or clinically inappropriate. (Panel Consensus)

46. Clinicians should:

    ■ Assess thoroughly each patient's pain mechanism in order to apply the most appropriate nerve block.

    ■ Screen patients for coexistent medical conditions, ability to understand risks of the proposed procedure, and ability to cooperate during the procedure.

    ■ Consider a block only if the person planning to do it is experienced and skillful, is prepared to deal with its immediate effects and side effects, and is able to provide follow-up assessment and treatment.

    ■ Use radiographic control for blocks when ease and safety depend on precise anatomic guidance. (Panel Consensus)

47. When a patient is painfree after neurolysis, opioids should not be stopped abruptly, lest a withdrawal syndrome be provoked. (B)

48. **The oncologic surgeon should be familiar with the interactions of chemotherapy, radiation therapy, and surgical interventions so that iatrogenic complications may be avoided or anticipated. (Panel Consensus)**

49. **The surgeon should recognize and treat characteristic pain syndromes that follow specific surgical procedures. (Panel Consensus)**

Introduction

Invasive nonpharmacologic interventions complement behavioral, physical, and drug therapies in a substantial minority of patients in whom these therapies alone do not control pain (see Figure 3). **With rare exception, noninvasive analgesic approaches should precede invasive palliative approaches.** Although radiotherapy and surgery can cure primary disease, they are discussed here in relation to pain relief only. Surgical procedures are useful in selected patients to debulk tumors and hence reduce symptoms of obstruction or compression. Anesthetic and neurosurgical methods can be used to ablate pain pathways or implant devices for drug delivery or electrical stimulation of neural structures. For any invasive therapy, the risks, availability of expertise and suitable support systems, and cost should be considered in addition to the apparent necessity or medical indication.

Radiation Therapy

Radiation therapy can relieve metastatic pain as well as symptoms from local extension of primary disease (Greenwald, Bonica, and Bergner, 1987). Over one-third of the practice of radiation therapy is palliative (Arcangeli, Micheli, Arcangeli, et al., 1989). The intent of any palliative treatment is to relieve pain quickly and maintain symptom control for the duration of the patient's life. Treatment is therefore tailored to the patient's clinical condition and overall prognosis (Lawton and Maher, 1991; Maher, Coia, Duncan, et al., 1992). Radiation therapy is complementary to analgesic drug therapies and may enhance their effectiveness because it directly targets the cause of pain.

In general, the larger the daily dose of radiation, the lower the total dose that can be administered because of limits to normal tissue tolerance. Proportionately more tumor cells are killed when the daily radiation dose is larger. A balance is required between the killing of tumor cells and the adverse radiation effects on normal tissues, which are largely a function of the daily dose. A number of different schedules have been developed that take into account specific tumor characteristics and the tolerance of normal tissues. The literature is divided regarding the optimal radiation schedule to achieve tumor regression (Hall, 1993; Thames, Withers, Peters, et al., 1982) and disease palliation (Price, Hoskin, Easton, et al., 1986) at either primary or metastatic sites. Generally, however, radiation treatment is planned in relation to clinical status.

The toxicity of radiation is determined by the structures included within the radiation portal, the dose per fraction, the total dose, and the radiation sensitivity of the tissues involved. **The desired dosage of radiation should be administered in the fewest fractions possible to promote patient comfort during and after treatment.** Radiation side effects are restricted to the radiation portal and can be classified as either acute, occurring during or immediately after the course of radiation therapy, or late, occurring months to years later. Acute radiation effects are more prominent with radiation schedules that deliver high total doses of radiation with small daily fractions; they generally begin at the end of the second week of therapy (Hall, 1993). Acute radiation effects, occurring primarily at skin and mucosal surfaces, usually consist of an inflammatory response such as skin erythema or pigmentation, or as mucositis. Acute reactions, however, are generally mild during palliative therapy schedules, which deliver high daily radiation doses over 1 to 2 weeks. Late radiation effects may arise without any preceding acute reactions. Fibrosis is the most common type of late radiation injury and can be observed in many types of tissue, including skin. Late effects are most prominent in tissues with limited regenerative capacity such as brain, peripheral nerves, and lungs. Because of the limited duration of patient survival, however, late effects are seldom seen after palliative radiotherapy.

Bone Metastases

Most patients referred for palliation of metastatic bone pain have primary tumors of the highest overall incidence: breast, prostate, or lung. Other neoplasms involving bone, such as myeloma, also respond to radiation. Regular followup should be provided to offer treatment of new symptoms or the use of other palliative techniques such as radiopharmaceuticals.

Plain radiographs are useful in detecting lytic or blastic lesions from bone metastases. Bone scintigraphy, however, is more sensitive than skeletal radiography for the detection of most bone metastases. Although 73 percent of patients in one series were asymptomatic when skeletal metastases were discovered by scintigraphy, 66 percent of these symptom-free patients ultimately experienced moderate to severe bone pain (Sherry, Greco, Johnson, et al., 1986a). In patients who experience bone pain and have normal bone scans, MRI may be a helpful diagnostic tool.

Indications for the radiation of bone metastases include pain relief and the prevention or promotion of healing of pathologic fractures. Spinal cord compression associated with vertebral collapse due to bony or epidural metastases requires emergent radiation therapy, sometimes in coordination with surgical intervention to preserve neurologic integrity (Bates, 1992). Orthopedic complications, including pathologic fracture and spinal cord compression, have been reported in 36 percent of breast cancer patients with skeletal metastases (Sherry, Greco, Johnson, et al., 1986b). Lytic lesions that are 2.5 cm or larger in weight-bearing bones or that cause a more than 50 percent loss of cortical bone place patients at high risk for pathologic fracture (Bates, 1992); patients with such lesions may benefit from prophylactic surgical fixation in conjunction with adjuvant irradiation.

Pain Relief With Localized Radiation Therapy. Radiation is commonly administered to a localized bone metastasis. An analysis of therapeutic results is complicated by variation in the location and extent of bone metastases, primary histology, individual differences (including patients' underlying medical conditions), and co-administered treatments. Concurrent analgesic use is frequently a confounding, poorly quantified variable in many accounts of pain control during local radiation of a metastasis. Most retrospective and prospective studies report that 75 percent or more of patients obtain relief from pain and that about half of those who achieve relief become pain-free (Nielsen, Munro, and Tannock, 1991). However, selection bias cannot be excluded; valid and reliable pain assessment instruments were not commonly used.

The literature is divided on appropriate fractionation (Blitzer, 1985; Hoskin, 1988; Tong, Gillick, and Hendrickson, 1982). Protracted regimens of more than 10 treatments may be more appropriate for patients with life expectancies of longer than 6 months to reduce potential late radiation effects or acute effects such as nausea if critical structures such as the stomach have to be included in the radiation field. For patients with a more limited life expectancy, radiation can be administered in fewer fractions, depending on the patient's clinical status (Lawton and Maher, 1991; Maher, Coia, Duncan, et al., 1992). These later regimens result in effective palliation in over 70 percent of patients at 3-months' followup, with negligible complications when radiation portals are localized (Arcangeli, Micheli, Arcangeli, et al., 1989; Bates, Yarnold, Blitzer, et al., 1992; Blitzer, 1985; Tong, Gillick, and Hendrickson, 1982).

Wide-Field Radiation Therapy. Hemibody irradiation, which can treat multiple disease sites, is particularly appropriate for diffuse bone pain. A single large fraction of 6 Gy to 8 Gy is administered to one half of the body. If necessary, the other half can be treated after a 3-week interval to allow for bone marrow recovery. With antiemetics and partial shielding to reduce lung exposure, toxicity occurs in fewer than 10 percent of patients, and 50 percent experience stabilization of disease at 1-year followup (Poulter, Cosmatos, Rubin, et al., 1992). Salazar, Rubin, Hendrickson, et al. (1986) reported that palliation was achieved in 73 percent of patients treated with hemibody irradiation, and pain recurrence was lower than that reported in an earlier uncontrolled study of the palliative effects of local radiotherapy (Tong, Gillick, and Hendrickson, 1982). This analysis is consistent with other reported studies of hemibody irradiation in which 50 percent of patients report at least partial pain relief within 48 hours of treatment with an eventual total response rate of 55 to 100 percent (Kuban, Schellhammer, and el-Mahdi, 1991; Salazar, Rubin, Hendrickson, et al., 1986).

Radiopharmaceuticals. Several radiopharmaceuticals have been used therapeutically. Iodine-131, used for the treatment of multiple bone metastases from thyroid cancer, results in bone scan evidence of response in 53 percent of patients (Maxon and Smith, 1990). Phosphorus-32-orthophosphate has provided partial or complete relief of pain in about 80 percent of patients with bone metastases from breast and prostate carcinoma (Silberstein, Elgazzar, and Kapilivsky, 1992). In an analysis of 18 published studies, strontium-89 was found to provide partial to complete pain relief for 65 percent (Silberstein, unpublished manuscript). For example, Silberstein and Williams (1985) reported a palliative response of 51 percent of patients, and Robinson, Spicer, Preston, et al. (1987) reported 80 to 89 percent palliative response. In these studies, analgesic use and activities of daily living were used as measures of palliation. Myelosuppression, manifested by approximately a 30 to 50 percent decline in leukocyte and platelet levels within 4 to 6 weeks, generally occurs in patients with either extensive disease or pretreatment peripheral cytopenia (Lewington, McEwan, Ackery, et al., 1991). Rhenium-186 and samarium-153 phosphonate chelates have demonstrated 65 to 80 percent efficacy in international clinical trials, with FDA approval pending (Maxon, Schroder, Thomas, et al., 1990; Turner, Claringbold, Hetherington, et al., 1989). These β-emitting radiopharmaceuticals, which require only a single intravenous injection, are used to relieve pain from widespread, osteoblastic skeletal metastases visualized with bone scintigraphy. If pain recurs, 50 percent of patients will respond to a second administration.

Plexopathy

Painful nerve compression or infiltration by a malignant tumor can sometimes be alleviated by radiation therapy. These primary tumors often require fractionated radiation therapy over 5 to 7 weeks in an attempt to secure local or regional control of the disease. Dosage is limited by the proximity of the tumor to radiosensitive structures, such as the spinal cord. Peripheral nerves, however, can tolerate higher doses.

Other Therapeutic Applications

Palliative radiation can be administered to any location of symptomatic primary or metastatic disease. Aggressive, sometimes protracted multimodality therapy may be given to patients with certain primary tumors, such as soft tissue sarcomas and carcinomas of the breast, lung, and rectum, to relieve both symptoms and to achieve control of advanced disease. Palliative radiation may also be given to metastatic lesions involving the brain, eye, skin, and soft tissue. Localized radiation may be used to treat lymph node involvement causing symptoms due to pressure on adjacent nerve roots and blood vessels. Intra-abdominal tumors may infiltrate the retroperitoneum and adjacent nerve roots or may cause local symptoms such as bowel obstruction. Although limited by the tolerance of the bowel to radiation, some tumor regression and symptomatic relief may be accomplished through fractionated radiation. Because the radiation tolerance of normal liver or kidney is even lower than that of bowel, treatment of pain due to capsular distention of either organ is rarely undertaken. Radiotherapy is generally not administered in these cases unless a trial of analgesic therapy and, when appropriate, chemotherapy has been unsuccessful. Symptomatic bleeding from endobronchial, cervical, and bladder tumors can often be stopped by external beam irradiation.

Brachytherapy

Brachytherapy involves the placement of a radioactive source within tissue to deliver localized radiation and is frequently applied to treat recurrent disease in an area previously treated by external beam radiation. Advantages include the sparing of critical structures close to the tumor, and brevity of treatment (hours to days). Difficulties primarily involve anatomic constraints on implant placement. Common applications include the endoluminal treatment of recurrent endobronchial and bile duct tumors, the intracavitary treatment of cervical and endometrial cancer, and interstitial implants in unresectable tumors with catheters or radioactive seeds. Occasionally, hyperthermia will be combined with either brachytherapy or external beam irradiation to relieve pain and other symptoms of recurrent disease originating from head and neck or breast cancers.

Anesthetic Techniques

Nerve Blocks_____

The possibility of controlling otherwise intractable pain by the relatively brief application of a local anesthetic or neurolytic agent makes neural blockade an attractive approach in selected patients. Published estimates of the percentage of all patients with cancer pain for whom nerve block procedures may appropriately be considered vary greatly. Variability in this estimate reflects evolution of the effectiveness of noninvasive therapies, interinstitutional differences in availability of clinicians with the necessary expertise, and access to alternative options such as spinal opioid therapy or neurosurgery (Bonica, Buckley, Moricca, et al., 1990). Allowing for vagueness in methods of arriving at published estimates, lack of uniformity in clinical conditions treated by neural blockade, and in reported clinical outcomes, it still appears that some 50 to 80 percent of patients who receive nerve blocks for cancer pain may benefit (Cousins and Bridenbaugh, 1987; Patt, 1993; Raj, 1992) (Table 19).

Local anesthetic such as lidocaine or bupivacaine is typically applied at an anatomically defined site to provide diagnostic information (e.g., whether the pain is somatic or visceral; whether it has a sympathetic mechanism). Prognostic injection assesses side effects such as hypotension and subjective sensations, including pain relief or unpleasant numbness, likely to result from a planned neurodestructive procedure. Although the lack of a desirable result from local anesthetic injection after proper needle placement generally predicts the failure of a neurolytic block, a promising result after local anesthetic injection does not guarantee the success of subsequent chemical destruction.

Therapeutic injections of a local anesthetic may provide relief that outlasts its pharmacologic action. Prolonged benefit may follow

Table 19. Nerve blocks

Purposes of Nerve Blocks

Diagnostic:	to determine source of pain (e.g., somatic nerve versus sympathetic pathways).
Therapeutic:	to treat painful conditions that respond to nerve blocks (e.g., celiac blocks for pain of pancreatic cancer).
Prognostic:	to predict outcome of permanent interventions such as infusions, neurolysis, and rhizotomy.
Preemptive:	to prevent painful sequelae of procedures that may cause phantom limb or causalgia.

injection of trigger points for myofascial pain—a procedure sufficiently simple, safe, and efficacious that it can be accomplished by many primary care providers. The injection of an anti-inflammatory corticoid with a local anesthetic into the spinal space or around nerve roots can reduce edema and irritation produced by tumor compression and provide analgesia for days to weeks. One or more cervical or lumbar sympathetic blocks may result in prolonged relief in patients whose cancer-related pain is sympathetically maintained. Sympathetic block performed during acute herpes zoster infection can immediately decrease pain, hasten resolution, and avert the development of postherpetic neuralgia, and should be considered as preemptive therapy for this debilitating sequel (Ferrer, 1989). The simpler technique of subcutaneous infiltration with local anesthetic and corticoid has also been reported to provide symptomatic relief for herpes zoster. When single sympathetic blocks produce only transient benefit, the placement of a catheter at the sympathetic ganglion (or the corresponding intraspinal segments or interpleural space) to enable continuous sympathetic blockade for days to weeks may produce sustained benefit.

Patient selection and timing of neural destruction for pain relief are based on the exhaustion of more conservative modalities, a lack of available, clinically superior options, and the availability of capable physician and support systems after the procedure. Nondestructive analgesic infusion techniques can preempt the need for neurolytic procedures. Therapeutic choices depend on patient and family preferences and the clinical judgment of their health care providers (Verrill, 1990).

Peripheral nerve destruction can be accomplished by the injection of ethanol, phenol, or other neurolytic agents at sites where a previous test injection of local anesthetic has produced pain relief. Whereas phenol induces warmth and then numbness, alcohol produces intense transient burning after injection and hence should be immediately preceded by local anesthetic injection. Small volumes of alcohol or phenol may be injected intrathecally to destroy nerve root function in a localized distribution. Approximately 60 percent of patients treated with intraspinal alcohol or phenol experience complete or near-complete relief of pain until death (Rodriquez-Bigas, Petrelli, Herrera, et al., 1991). **When a patient is painfree after neurolysis, opioids should not be stopped abruptly, lest a withdrawal syndrome be provoked.** Complications including paresis, paralysis, and bowel or bladder dysfunction affect 0.5 to 2 percent of patients treated with intraspinal alcohol or phenol (Gerbershagen, 1981). An epidural injection of phenol (or alcohol, according to some reports) can accomplish the same goal; however, the targeting of the injectate is less precise, the neurolytic effects take place over a more diffuse area than that affected by the intrathecal route, and the technique is less well established than intrathecal injection (Salmon, Finch, Lovegrove, et al., 1992).

Neurolytic sympathetic blockade is useful to relieve pain in the arm, head and neck (stellate ganglion), or leg (lumbar sympathetic block), as well as to interrupt the visceral afferent pain pathways mediating pain in the pancreas and other upper abdominal organs (celiac block) or in the pelvis (hypogastric block). Side effects of celiac block include transient hypotension and diarrhea; complications (less likely with radiologic guidance) include paraplegia or less severe radicular weakness or numbness, intrarenal injection and damage, retroperitoneal hematoma, and failure of ejaculation (Ischia, Ischia, Polati, et al., 1992; van Dongen and Crul, 1991). Four-fifths or more of patients with pancreatic or other abdominal cancers derive pain relief from celiac block, usually lasting until death (Brown, Bulley, and Quiel, 1987; Eisenberg, Carr, and Chalmers, unpublished manuscript; Mercandante, 1993). Even when relief is incomplete, patients may appreciate the ability to lower their opioid dosage and by doing so reduce drowsiness and constipation. It thus appears reasonable to consider early celiac neurolytic block for patients with a short life expectancy and pain from pancreatic cancer (Mercadante, 1993). A recently reported technique for refractory chest wall tumor pain is interpleural blockade, which uses long-term local anesthetic infusion or single-dose phenol (Lema, Myers, de Leon-Casasola, et al., 1992).

Neurolytic blockade of peripheral nerves should be reserved for instances in which other therapies (palliative irradiation, TENS, pharmacotherapy) are ineffective, poorly tolerated, or clinically inappropriate. Suitable targets for this approach include intercostal nerves at the site of painful tumor, after maximal doses of radiation and systemic analgesics, or nerves of the head and neck (e.g., gasserian ganglion). Pain recurrence due to neuritis is common because an alcohol-damaged nerve regenerates over weeks to months. If the mechanism of pain is partial or complete denervation, this will not be corrected (and may potentially be worsened) by further chemical damage to the nerve.

Pain that is diffuse (e.g., from multiple bony metastases) may respond to chemical ablation of the pituitary, which is accomplished by alcohol administered through a needle advanced transnasally until its tip rests in the pituitary fossa (see also Neurosurgery, below). Pain relief by this intervention may be rapid and striking, while ascending nociceptive pathways remain unharmed. Pain relief has been reported in about two-thirds of patients, whether or not the primary tumor is hormone dependent (Takeda, Fujii, Uki, et al., 1983). Complications include headache, persistent leakage of CSF, coma, and cranial nerve palsies, all of which occur at a frequency of 5 percent or less (Cook, Campbell, and Puddy, 1984). Diabetes insipidus is a predictable side effect of complete pituitary ablation.

Technical aspects of the above procedures are beyond the scope of this guideline and are well described in a number of recent monographs (Abram, 1989; Charlton, 1986; Cousins and Bridenbaugh, 1987; Swerdlow, 1987). Complications associated with local anesthetic nerve blocks, catheter implants, neurostimulator implants, thermal ablations, and neurolytic injection have been reported (Cousins and Bridenbaugh, 1987; Melzack and Wall, 1989; Raj, 1992). Serious side effects including hemorrhage, infection, unexpected nerve damage, pneumothorax, and cardiorespiratory arrest are rare but nonetheless mandate resuscitative skills and close short-term followup.

Because of the appeal of nerve blocks for use in intractable pain and their potential for harm as well as benefit, clinicians should:

- Assess thoroughly each patient's pain mechanism, in order to apply the most appropriate block.

- Screen patients according to coexistent medical conditions (e.g., coagulopathy); ability to understand risks of the proposed procedure (e.g., paresis or incontinence); and ability to cooperate during the procedure (e.g., not move).

- Consider a block only if the person planning to do it is experienced and skillful; prepared to deal with its immediate effects and side effects (e.g., hypotension, respiratory depression, or paralysis); and able to provide followup assessment and treatment.

- Use radiographic control for blocks when ease and safety depend on the precise identification of landmarks.

Catheter Placement for Drug Delivery

Temporary spinal or epidural catheter placement is normally undertaken by specialists trained to recognize possible complications (e.g., opioid-induced respiratory depression or hypotension or sensorimotor blockade due to local anesthetic) and able to deal with these promptly and effectively. The need for dosage titration and coordination of spinal with systemic medications and nonmedical therapies requires that the catheter be placed within the framework of multidisciplinary continuing care. Because identical materials and methods are often used for percutaneous epidural catheter placement for cancer pain and for acute postoperative pain control, anesthesiologists typically perform these techniques and their specific followup. Factors to consider are presented in Table 12. The placement of catheters other than spinal ones, such as for drug infusion into interpleural or paravertebral areas, is uncommon, and few data other than case reports are available.

Percutaneous electrical stimulation for the relief of otherwise refractory cancer pain has likewise not yet been evaluated in controlled trials. Case reports—limited essentially to the percutaneous insertion of spinal cord electrodes for dorsal column stimulation—tend to focus on details of the method, to use nonuniform patient selection criteria, and to use heterogeneous pain assessment methods and followup duration. Not all experience is favorable (Meglio, Cioni, and Rossi, 1989). Hence, as Miles and colleagues wrote nearly 20 years ago, "At this stage it seems sensible to concentrate effort on evaluating the method rather than on encouraging widespread and possibly indiscriminate use of what is an expensive use and relatively unproven technique" (Miles, Lipton, Hayward, et al., 1974).

Neurosurgery

Neurosurgical procedures for the relief of pain include neuroablation, implantation of drug infusion systems, and neuroaugmentation. Published estimates of the percentage of patients who require neurosurgical procedures to control cancer-related pain vary but are nearly all fewer than 10 percent. Nevertheless, long-standing clinical experience supports a view that neurosurgical intervention is appropriate for patients in whom more conservative treatment is neither tolerated nor effective (or is unlikely to be effective) and for whom the expertise and followup care are available. The choice of procedure is based on the location and type of pain (somatic, visceral, deafferentation), the general condition of the patient, the life expectancy, and the expertise available.

There is no simple, entirely safe procedure to alleviate cancer-related pain. Depending on the clinical setting and procedure, the risks of neurosurgical operation include new pain symptoms from nerve damage at the site of incision or nerve division, recurrence of pain after a transiently successful result, and postoperative neurologic impairment. These risks must be balanced against an ideal possible outcome of abolition of pain with little or no need for medication. In a particular clinical situation, a lack of personnel with experience in carrying out and following up other invasive therapies may warrant greater reliance on neurosurgical options (e.g., cordotomy instead of epidural catheter for pain of pelvic tumor). Because appropriate patient selection is essential, each proposed neurosurgical intervention is best reviewed by a team of oncologists, pain specialists, psychotherapists, and neurosurgeons.

The following discussion addresses only procedures that are in general use and for which reported results can be meaningfully assessed. Classic (White and Sweet, 1969) and recent textbooks and monographs provide current reviews of all of these procedures (Bonica, 1990; Gybels and Sweet, 1989; Patt, 1993).

Neuroablation

Peripheral Neurectomy. Currently, peripheral neurectomy for the control of cancer pain has largely been supplanted by other techniques, such as neuraxial opioid infusion or lytic nerve block. Multilevel neurectomy for chest wall pain is indicated when a discrete pain-producing lesion can be demonstrated to involve several intercostal nerves (Arbit, Galicich, Burt, et al., 1989). Neurectomy may also be effective in alleviating pain originating from a paraspinal tumor that involves a nerve or nerves at or distal to the neural foramen; it is often performed at the time of an operation on the spine (e.g., anterior or posterolateral vertebrectomy). Cranial neurectomies have selected indications in neuralgias resulting from cancer. The trigeminal and glossopharyngeal nerves can be ablated by radiofrequency lesions created by electrodes placed in either the foramen ovale (gasserian ganglion) or the jugular foramen or by chemical neurolysis at the gasserian ganglion (Giorgi and Broggi, 1984; Ischia, Luzzani, and Polati, 1990; Sweet, 1976).

Dorsal Rhizotomy. Selective ablation of the dorsal nerve root reduces nociceptive perception in the affected area and spares motor function. Multilevel dorsal rhizotomy of all roots supplying an extremity leads to a functionless limb. The likelihood of this impairment is lessened by sparing one dorsal root. In practice, this procedure is considered only for localized pain in the trunk or abdomen or, rarely, for an extremity that is functionless preoperatively (Arbit, Galicich, Burt, et al., 1989; Sindou, Fischer, Goutelle, et al., 1981). Dorsal rhizotomy can be accomplished by chemical neurolysis with radiographic guidance to place the tip of an infusion catheter at the precise segment within the epidural space. Surgical rhizotomy may be necessary if expertise in chemical neurolysis is unavailable or if it has been tried unsuccessfully.

Anterolateral Cordotomy (Spinal Tractotomy). Anterolateral cordotomy is an ablative procedure aimed at the pain-conducting tracts in the anterolateral quadrant of the spinal cord. Cordotomy provides selective loss of pain and temperature perception several segments below and contralateral to the segment at which the lesion is placed. Anterolateral cordotomy is effective for unilateral, mainly somatic pain below the midcervical dermatomes (Ischia, Ischia, Luzzani, et al., 1985; Lahuerta, Lipton, and Wells, 1985). For visceral pain or bilateral pain, bilateral cordotomies may be required (Amano, Kawamura, Tanikawa, et al., 1991). Most cordotomies are currently done with the patient under local anesthesia by the percutaneous route under fluoroscopic guidance, and the lesion is created by radiofrequency. The percutaneous approach avoids risks of open operation and anesthesia in patients in poor medical condition.

Open cordotomies require a laminectomy and are most frequently performed at the low cervical or upper thoracic spine. Open cordotomy may benefit patients in whom a percutaneous procedure has failed, those who cannot cooperate because of severe pain or confusion, those at risk for respiratory compromise, or those with bilateral pain in whom a bilateral, high cervical cordotomy carries additional risk of neurologic impairment. Potential complications include unmasking of dysesthetic pain; bladder, bowel, and sexual dysfunction; ataxia; paresis; and sleep apnea (Lahuerta, Lipton, and Wells, 1985; Tasker, 1988).

Commissural Myelotomy. Commissural myelotomy disrupts pain-conducting fibers as well as a polysynaptic pain pathway that runs through the center of the spinal cord. Indications for myelotomy are bilateral and midline pelvic or perineal pain (Adams, Lippert, and Hosobuchi, 1988; van Roost and Gybels, 1989). The procedure may produce sphincter or motor dysfunction. Open myelotomy involves a multilevel laminectomy and exposure of the appropriate lumbar or sacral segments of the spinal cord. By use of an operating microscope, a midline incision is made and the spinal cord is divided vertically (Gildenberg, 1984). A cervicomedullary junction (extralemniscal) myelotomy that is performed stereotactically with CT guidance, local anesthesia, and intraoperative physiologic assessment can achieve pain relief over wide areas of the body including midline structures (Schvarcz, 1978). Potential complications include temporary dysesthesia and limb apraxia (Gildenberg, 1984).

Hypophysectomy. Surgical and chemical (stereotactic transsphenoidal) hypophysectomy are similar procedures that each offer a 40 to 70 percent likelihood of pain relief (Levin, Katz, Benson, et al., 1980). The mechanism by which pain relief is achieved is unknown, but it is not related directly to the expected fall in the pituitary hormone levels, because pain relief is achieved in hormonally independent and dependent tumors (Katz and Levin, 1977; Lipton, Miles, Williams, et al., 1978; Takeda, Fujii, Uki, et al., 1983). The clearest clinical indication is for bilateral or diffuse bone pain from metastatic disease that has failed to respond to all other hormonal, radiation, or medical therapies. Hormone replacement therapy is needed to replace pituitary secretion. Potential complications include endocrine deficits, damage to the optic nerves or oculomotor apparatus from the injected chemical agent, and CSF leakage (Cook, Campbell, and Puddy, 1984; Lahuerta, Lipton, Miles, et al., 1985; Lipton, Miles, Williams, et al., 1978).

Neuraxial Opioid Infusion

In properly selected patients, intraspinal or intraventricular infusions of opioids have the advantage of producing profound analgesia without motor, sensory, or sympathetic blockade (Behar, Magora, Olshwang, et al., 1979; Bullingham, McQuay, and Moore, 1982). See Chapter 3 and also the section on catheter placement in this chapter for a discussion of intraspinal and intraventricular routes of administration.

Neuroaugmentation

Interest in endogenous pain control systems as a therapeutic target began over 20 years ago in the context of the contemporaneous discoveries of the positive reinforcing quality of electric self-stimulation of the brain in animals and humans. Profound analgesia without drugs was reported in laboratory animals during electrical stimulation of the brain stem (Reynolds, 1969; Yaksh and Rudy, 1976). These effects appear to depend on the body's own opioids, endorphins. Since then, electrical stimulation for cancer pain control has been directed at deep brain structures such as the periaqueductal and periventricular grey areas (Meyerson, Boethius, and Carlsson, 1978; Young and Brechner, 1986), the limbic system (Gol, 1967), and other more superficial sites such as the pituitary gland (Yanagida, Suwa, Trouwborst, et al., 1988). Evaluation of the efficacy of electrical stimulation ("neuroaugmentation") of deep brain structures for cancer pain relief, as for many other modalities, is difficult because of scanty descriptions of patients' diagnoses and limited pain assessment and followup, as well as the relatively few patients treated in this fashion compared with much larger numbers treated, e.g., with pharmacotherapy. Nonetheless, the few descriptive, uncontrolled published studies report partial or complete pain relief in 27 to 76 percent of patients treated by neuroaugmentation (Meglio and Cioni, 1982; Meyerson, 1982; Young and Brechner, 1986). Published results of spinal cord stimulation for cancer pain relief are less encouraging. Meglio and others (Meglio, Cioni, and Rossi, 1989) reported, in a series of 109 patients treated for pain relief by means of spinal cord stimulation, that none of the 11 who had cancer pain derived any clinical benefit, in contrast to favorable responses observed in patients with vasculopathic pain or postherpetic neuralgia. Similarly, others (North, 1993; Gybels, 1993; Marchand, 1993) have found spinal cord stimulation useful to treat chronic pain if not due to malignancy and only anecdotal observations support the success of this modality in patients with cancer-related pain (Miles, Lipton, Hayward, et al., 1974; Nittner, 1980; Raj, 1992).

Surgery

Operations for the curative excision or palliative debulking of a tumor have the potential to reduce pain, improve prognosis, and even to achieve long-term, symptom-free survival. On the other hand, a tumor may be recognized to be unresectable at the time of operation. These perioperative dilemmas provoke anxiety in patients and their families, who worry not only about mortality but also about possible survival at the expense of function or loss of body parts. This anxiety may worsen pain.

The surgeon's response to these issues can help to create a sense of personal comfort, to reduce the feelings of loss of control in patients confronted with a loss of autonomy, if not life itself, and to foster a clear understanding of the pain- and tumor-control goals of the surgical procedure and of how the procedure relates to other aspects of treatment.

Postoperatively, the patient is often left with major changes in anatomy and physiology (e.g., laryngectomy, colostomy) that require further rehabilitation and continued attention to pain control. The surgeon should convey the nature and implications of the surgical intervention to the other members of the patient's management team and should continue in an advocacy role throughout the patient's course of care (Dunphy, 1976).

Continuing surgical care is ideally provided in the context of an interdisciplinary approach with an attempt to avoid fragmentation and duplication. A vital part of surgical care for malignant disease is followup to contribute to improving quality of life, particularly the reduction of pain and suffering, to give assistance in rehabilitation, and to provide psychological support for the patient (O'Young and McPeek, 1987). The patient and family seek assurance that the surgeon will not abandon them postoperatively and will be available for acute and chronic pain control.

Surgical Management of Pain Due To Primary or Metastatic Tumor

Pain control is usually a secondary goal when curative tumor excision is performed. In contrast, when surgery is palliative because the tumor is unresectable, pain control is frequently the operative indication. Cancer pain may arise through a variety of mechanisms that are amenable to relief by surgery. During curative or palliative procedures surgeons should use techniques to limit the development of chronic neuropathic pain such as nerve-sparing incisions, avoidance of ischemia, and careful dissection around nerves. **The oncologic surgeon**

should be familiar with the interactions of chemotherapy, radiation therapy, and surgical interventions so that iatrogenic complications may be avoided or anticipated (e.g., multiple fistulas resulting from bowel resection performed after radiation).

Surgical procedures should proceed within a framework of basic surgical oncology principles that relate to both curative and palliative surgery. Among these is the fundamental principle that the first resection offers the best opportunity for cure. Occasionally, an anatomic structure will need to be removed during this initial curative procedure to achieve a resection margin free of tumor. Careful preoperative and intraoperative weighing of the benefits of potentially curative procedures versus the risks of chronic pain and disability should be done with the patient preoperatively and confirmed by the surgeon intraoperatively.

The second principle is that even outstanding radiotherapy generally will not improve an inadequate surgical procedure. Depending on the natural history of a specific tumor system and anatomic constraints, postoperative radiotherapy can enhance local tumor control in patients with microscopically positive margins. However, radiotherapy may not provide long-term durable control of residual macroscopic gross malignant disease. Therefore, a surgical procedure undertaken for pain control is also most effective and durable if all gross disease can be resected. Short- and long-term pain control may be enhanced with postoperative radiotherapy. As a corollary to this principle, simple tumor debulking generally does not provide durable palliation for most patients. Growth of the residual tumor is sufficient to cause a rapid recurrence of painful symptoms. In such patients, radiotherapy alone may provide better palliation than an incomplete resection with its attendant pain.

The third principle is that local tumor recurrence is not always the harbinger of disseminated disease. For example, local recurrence of soft tissue sarcoma or colorectal carcinoma does not always behave in this manner. Consequently, some patients with local recurrence can still be cured, depending on their underlying disease. Such patients may be best served by a second resection aimed at cure, perhaps incorporating radiotherapy, rather than a less aggressive palliative procedure solely for pain control.

The fourth principle is that the timing of a surgical intervention for pain control is important. Understanding the natural history of a tumor system includes an awareness of the potential of a given tumor type for local invasion as well as tumor-specific patterns of metastasis. This addresses the issue of prospective palliation in which the effectiveness of surgical pain control may be maximized if undertaken before the onset of symptoms. For example, stabilizing a long bone with lytic metastases where fracture is likely or decompressing a spinal canal to prevent impending paralysis or to relieve tumor nerve root entrapment may be most helpful as a timely intervention before the development of irreversible symptoms. This is in contrast to the asymptomatic patient with a recurrent, widely metastatic carcinoma of the colon that may eventually cause intestinal obstruction. In these instances, it may be better to monitor the patient closely for the development of symptoms rather than intervene early and disrupt the quality of life.

Pain as a Consequence of Operation

Surgical procedures can cause several different forms of pain, including incisional pain. Depending on the resection and the specific tissues removed, patients may experience deep wound pain that may be more difficult to control. Finally, many patients may experience a variety of chronic pain syndromes after surgery (see Table 5). Some of these may not emerge until weeks or months after discharge. **The surgeon should recognize and treat characteristic pain syndromes that follow specific surgical procedures (e.g., mastectomy, nephrectomy, etc.).**

Careful surgical technique frequently can ameliorate the severity of postoperative pain. Gentle tissue handling; use of nerve- or vessel-sparing procedures; avoidance of tissue ischemia; careful neurolysis, performed as needed with a dissecting microscope; and selection of non-muscle-splitting incisions can contribute to less painful surgery and recovery.

In the postoperative period, the surgeon should encourage the full use of the pain-control armamentarium. The management of patients with acute pain such as that caused by pathologic fracture, surgery, or diagnostic treatment procedures is described in detail elsewhere (Acute Pain Management Guideline Panel, 1992).

The surgeon should assess the quality of postoperative pain control by frequent, direct patient contact. The surgeon without expertise in pain management should seek consultative help, particularly for the treatment of special populations. An integrated multidisciplinary pain control approach will maximize the usefulness of surgery as an adjunct of pain control in the patient with cancer.

6 Procedure-Related Pain in Adults and Children

Recommendations

50. For patients of all ages, interventions for managing procedure-related pain and distress should take into account the type of procedure, the anticipated level of pain, and such individual factors as age and emotional and physical condition. (B)

51. Sedation should be considered for painless procedures that require patient cooperation in remaining still, particularly for children under 6 years of age and for cognitively impaired patients. (B)

52. Conscious sedation for procedural pain should be done in a manner that emphasizes safety and monitoring. (B)

Patients with cancer undergo painful procedures for diagnosis, therapy, and supportive care, including lumbar puncture, bone marrow aspiration, and biopsy. Although venipunctures, insertion of intravenous catheters, and intramuscular injections are less invasive, less painful procedures, their frequency and repetition become a major source of distress and apprehension. For aggressive treatment protocols, multiple invasive procedures may be performed weekly or daily.

Children with cancer consider painful procedures to be the most difficult part of having cancer, and frequent repetition of procedures does not desensitize them to the distress (Fowler-Kerry, 1990; Weekes and Savedra, 1988). No published studies have focused on the reactions of adults to frequent and cumulative procedures, but some adults may be able to cope because of their greater cognitive ability and life experience in dealing with adversity and stress. Nevertheless, what is painful for a child or adolescent is also likely to be painful for an adult, especially when already stressed by the diagnosis of a potentially fatal illness. For all cancer patients, then, intervention for suffering should include concern for and management of the pain and distress associated with procedures.

Much of the data available on the management of procedure-related pain comes from studies on children with cancer and addresses nonpharmacologic management. For these guidelines, relevant data on cognitive-behavioral management in children were extrapolated to adults when there were no studies with adult patients.

Managing Procedure-Related Pain

Painless procedures (such as CT scanning, MRI positioning for radiotherapy, and ultrasonic examination) that require patients to lie still, often on a cold, hard surface, may be frightening and indirectly provoke pain and distress. For patients older than 5 years, preparatory education about the sensations and surroundings the patient will experience (Johnson, Rice, Fuller, et al., 1978) and the use of hypnosis, distraction, imagery (Katz, Kellerman, and Ellenberg, 1987; Zeltzer, Altman, Cohen, et al., 1990), and relaxation (Pfaff, Smith, and Gowan, 1989) may decrease distress and facilitate coping with the procedure. **Sedatives, including oral chloral hydrate, pentobarbital, and midazolam (Sievers, Yee, Foley, et al., 1991), may be appropriate for painless procedures that require patient cooperation in remaining still, particularly for children under 6 years of age and for cognitively impaired patients.** Because pharmacologic sedation may result in the loss of protective reflexes, patients must be closely monitored (American Academy of Pediatrics Committee on Drugs, 1992). Intrinsically painful procedures may exacerbate ongoing cancer-related pain, and supplemental analgesia may be required (Table 20).

Plans for managing pain associated with painful procedures should address several questions:

■ Why is the procedure being performed?

■ What is the expected intensity of pain?

■ What is the expected duration of pain?

■ What is the expected intensity of anxiety?

■ What is the expected duration of anxiety?

■ How often will the procedure be repeated?

■ How do parents think their child will react? What reaction do adults predict for themselves?

■ What is the meaning of the procedure for the patient and the family?

Pharmacologic Strategies for Procedural Pain

The needs of the individual and the type of procedure to be performed shape the pharmacologic approach to managing procedure-related pain. Because children have special needs, the practitioner's expertise and experience with children are key to successful therapy. For all patients, an opioid or a local anesthetic is needed to

Table 20. General principles of management for painful procedures

General considerations

Treat anticipated procedure-related pain prophylactically.

Patients benefit from predictability as to time, frequency, and "clustering" of procedures, with an identified block of time when no procedures are to be performed, barring emergencies.

Be attentive to the environment and to privacy. For children, a room other than the child's room should be used whenever possible. Environmental factors, such as cold or crowded rooms or "beepers" on machines, can escalate distress (Fowler-Kerry, 1990; Hester, 1989).

Before beginning the procedure, manage preexisting pain as well as possible.

Tailor treatment options to the patient's and the family's needs and preferences, to the procedure, and to the context.

Integrate pharmacologic and nonpharmacologic options in a complementary style.

After the procedure, review with the patient and family their experiences and perceptions about the effectiveness of pain management strategies.

Psychological preparation of the patient

Provide adequate preparation of the patient and family. For children, discuss with the child and parents what can be expected and how the child might respond.

Procedural considerations

For procedures that will be repeated, maximize treatment for the pain and anxiety of the first procedure to minimize anxiety before subsequent procedures.

Ensure the competency of the person performing the procedure and the timeliness of the procedure (Zeltzer, Altman, Cohen, et al., 1990).

Minimize delays to prevent escalation of pain and anxiety (Fowler-Kerry, 1990).

Provide monitoring and resuscitative equipment if drugs are used for sedation. Facilities, equipment, and trained personnel to manage emergencies (e.g., vomiting, inadequate ventilation, and anaphylaxis) should be immediately available (American Academy of Pediatrics Committee on Drugs, 1992; American Nurses Association, 1992).

Nonpharmacologic interventions

For children, allow parents to be with the child during the procedure, if parents choose to remain. The presence of a parent is a source of great comfort for the child (Bauchner, Waring, and Vinci, 1991). The parent's knowledge of the child can be valuable. Parents should be taught what to do, where to be, and what to say to help their child through the procedure. Parents should not be asked to restrain the child during the procedure.

For adults, the presence of a supportive friend or relative may be helpful (Puntillo, 1990). Elicit the patient's preferences in this regard.

Infants can benefit from sensory motor interventions (e.g., using a pacifier, touching, and patting) (Campos, 1989; NAACOG Committee on Practice, 1991). Potentially effective cognitive-behavioral strategies for older children

**Table 20. General principles of management for
painful procedures, continued**

include distraction techniques such as music (Ryan, 1989), coping skills (Siegel and Peterson, 1981), hypnosis (Kuttner, 1988; Olness, 1981; Zeltzer and LeBaron, 1982), play therapy (Ellerton, Caty, and Ritchie, 1985), and thought stopping (Ross, 1984). Physical agents include TENS therapy (Eland, 1989) and counterirritants such as ice (Zeltzer, Altman, Cohen, et al., 1990). Cognitive-behavioral interventions that have been effective in reducing procedural pain or analgesic use in adults include imagery (Horan, Laying, and Pursell, 1976) and hypnosis (Reeves, Redd, Storm, et al., 1983), and sensory and procedural information (Reading, 1982). Many of these methods, including the provision of preparatory information, hypnosis, thought stopping, and counterirritation, may also be useful for adults. For all ages, choice should be based on the patient's preference, personality, and coping style.

Pharmacologic interventions

If possible, administer pharmacologic agents by a painless route (e.g., oral, transdermal, or intravenous). If parenteral agents are necessary and the patient does not have intravenous access, a single injection may be preferable to multiple attempts at insertion of an intravenous catheter.

reduce the pain. Anxiolytics (i.e., medications for the relief of anxiety) and sedatives are used specifically to reduce anxiety before and during the procedure, but if used alone (i.e., without an analgesic), they may blunt the behavioral response without relieving the pain. Patients who have built up a tolerance to opioids or benzodiazepines may need much higher initial doses than those given in Table 21.

Cardiovascular, hemodynamic, neurologic, or pulmonary instability are not absolute contraindications to systemic analgesia, but careful titration and monitoring should be provided. No agent should be used unless the clinician understands the proper technique of administration, the proper dosage, contraindications, side effects, and treatment of overdose. The use of systemic analgesics and sedatives should be approached differently in infants younger than 6 months of age (see Chapter 7).

The mixture of meperidine, promethazine, and chlorpromazine is not recommended even though commonly given intramuscularly for painful procedures in children. The efficacy of this mixture is controversial; disadvantages include the need for painful intramuscular injection and the prolonged sedation associated with its use (Nahata, Clotz, and Krogg, 1985).

Nitrous oxide, ketamine, thiopental, propofol, and methohexital can also be used as part of the pharmacologic strategy if trained personnel and appropriate monitoring procedures are available (Zeltzer, Jay, and Fisher, 1989). Administered by a mask or tent, nitrous oxide is a potent, short-acting inhalant analgesic that has been

Table 21. Pharmacologic agents for management of procedural pain

Local anesthetics

These agents may be administered by local infiltration or topical application. For topical use, an eutectic mixture of local anesthetics (EMLA) is efficacious in use with procedures and is now available in the United States (Kapelushnik, Koren, Solh, et al., 1990). When EMLA is used as a local anesthetic, it should be applied 60 to 90 minutes before the procedure.

Opioids

These drugs can be given via the intravenous or oral route. The intravenous route has the advantage of rapid effect and ease of titration. Intravenous opioids can be given in increments (e.g., 0.03 to 0.05 mg per kg of **morphine** every 5 minutes for children and other patients who weigh less than 50 kg, or 2 to 4 mg of morphine every 5 minutes for adults and children who weigh more than 50 kg) and titrated to analgesic effect (Schechter, Weisman, Rosenblum, et al., 1990). Oral opioids can be used when close and rapid titration to effect is not required.

Other opioids may be used instead of morphine. **Meperidine** is suitable for brief, titrated dosing but not for prolonged use. Intravenous **fentanyl** may be used in small doses (25-μg increments, or 0.5 μg/kg for patients who weigh 50 kg or less). If given slowly in increments, the risk of chest wall rigidity is extremely small, but if it occurs, it should be managed immediately by the administration of a rapid-onset muscle relaxant and supporting ventilation. Transdermal **fentanyl** is not recommended for this indication because it requires on average 14 hours to reach peak application after administration (Varvel, Shafer, Hwang, et al., 1989).

Benzodiazepines

These agents can be given orally, intravenously, or transmucosally and provide anxiolysis, skeletal muscle relaxation, and in higher doses, amnesia. After opioids, intravenous benzodiazepines are given in increments and titrated to sedative effect (Sievers, Yee, Foley, et al., 1991; Zeltzer, Altman, Cohen, et al., 1990). Unlike **diazepam, midazolam** does not cause pain and local sclerosis when given intravenously (Zeltzer, Altman, Cohen, et al., 1990). For adults, **midazolam** is traditionally titrated in increments of about 0.5 mg. Benzodiazepines provide sedation, not analgesia, and hence, they often are used with opioids for painful procedures. If the combination of opioid plus benzodiazepine is used, the risk of respiratory depression is increased significantly, and careful titration and monitoring are required, particularly in the elderly.

Barbiturates

These drugs provide excellent sedation. They have no analgesic effects and are used with analgesics for painful procedures. Some patients may have paradoxical reactions, and for most patients, the sedation persists for many hours after the procedure is completed (Zeltzer, Jay, and Fisher, 1989). As with benzodiazepines, close observation for respiratory depression is essential, particularly when the intravenous route is used or if an opioid is coadministered.

used for procedural pain and in the treatment of refractory pain in the terminally ill. A significant drawback is the high degree of room air contamination, making occupational exposure a serious concern. Thus, although nitrous oxide may be valuable, its use should be limited to situations in which appropriate environmental adaptations, trained personnel, and monitoring procedures are in place (Miser, Ayesh, Broda, et al., 1988). General anesthesia is appropriate in certain situations (Zeltzer, Altman, Cohen, et al., 1990) such as when a young child must undergo a painful procedure.

Sedation for Procedural Pain

Skilled supervision is necessary whenever systemic pharmacologic agents are used for conscious sedation (i.e., the patient maintains a response to verbal and physical stimuli). At any site where painful procedures may be performed, patient-size-appropriate resuscitative equipment and resuscitative drugs should be immediately available to treat promptly any untoward effects. **When conscious sedation is used, at least one health care professional who is well trained in airway management and advanced life support should be available.** Patients should not eat or drink before procedures that use conscious sedation.

During such procedures, a health care professional not involved in performing the procedure or restraining the patient should monitor the patient. Monitoring includes frequent assessment of heart rate, respiratory rate and effort, blood pressure, and level of consciousness. Continuous pulse oximetry to measure arterial oxygen saturation is strongly encouraged because visual observation of cyanosis is not sensitive to level of oxygen saturation. Guidelines from the American Academy of Pediatrics (1992) emphasize the importance of vigilant monitoring during conscious sedation:

> *The caveat that loss of consciousness should be unlikely is a particularly important aspect of the definition of conscious sedation, and the drugs and techniques used should carry a margin of safety wide enough to render unintended loss of consciousness highly unlikely. Since the patient who receives conscious sedation may progress into a state of deep sedation and obtundation, the practitioner should be prepared to increase the level of vigilance corresponding to that necessary for deep sedation. (p. 1112)*

After the procedure, monitoring should continue until the patient is fully awake and has resumed the former level of function. Discharged patients should be accompanied by an adult for a time at least as long as two half-lives of the agents used (e.g., at least 6 hours for morphine). These patients should be advised not to drive an automobile or operate dangerous machinery until it is likely that all medication effects are resolved (usually 24 to 48 hours). Documentation of the monitoring during the procedure, observation before discharge, and discharge instructions should be part of the patient's permanent record.

In contrast to conscious sedation, deep sedation (i.e., when the patient is not responsive to verbal or physical stimuli) is equivalent to general anesthesia and should be performed only under controlled circumstances by a professional trained in its use and skilled in airway management and advanced life support. Reference to specific published guidelines is recommended (e.g., in particular, American Academy of Pediatrics, 1985, 1992; American Nurses Association, 1991).

Despite careful titration of sedative doses, individual responses are variable, and patients may occasionally have respiratory compromise or loss of airway reflexes. Because respiratory depression is strongly related to the degree of sedation, stimulation of the patient, and administration of small doses of naloxone (e.g., 0.04-mg doses for patients weighing 40 kg or more, or 0.5 to 2 μg/kg for patients weighing less than 40 kg), may be adequate to reverse mild degrees of hypoventilation (Schechter, Weisman, Rosenblum, et al., 1990). Assisted ventilation by bag and mask or (ultimately) by endotracheal intubation and repetitive naloxone dosing may be required to reverse severe degrees of respiratory depression. If such depression does occur, the patient should be observed until well after the naloxone effect has worn off (usually after 1 hour).

Additional Pain Management Strategies for Lumbar Puncture and Bone Marrow Aspiration

For lumbar punctures, local anesthetics are used, although efficacy in infants is controversial. Young children and some older children and adults benefit from a benzodiazepine. Supplementation with opioids is helpful for some patients, especially when difficulty in performing the procedure is anticipated. Patients over 5 years of age, who can effectively use cognitive and behavioral coping skills, may prefer not to use sedatives or opioids (Zeltzer, Altman, Cohen, et al., 1990).

Management for bone marrow aspirations and biopsies includes the use, along with local anesthesia, of either general anesthesia or conscious sedation with benzodiazepines and opioids. Adequate time is necessary for the local anesthetic agent to have full effect.

In children, nonpharmacologic methods with demonstrated efficacy for lumbar punctures and bone marrow aspirations and biopsies include hypnosis (Zeltzer and LeBaron, 1982); thought stopping (Ross, 1984); and a multidimensional psychological intervention that includes a breathing exercise, reinforcement, imagery, behavioral rehearsal, and filmed modeling (Jay, Elliott, Ozolins, et al., 1985). These strategies alone, however, often do not reduce pain sufficiently.

In addressing procedure-related pain, clinicians should consider the nature of the procedure (invasive or noninvasive), the degree of pain expected, and the needs of the patient in the development of a plan that emphasizes prevention of pain before the procedure. Further, especially in children, followup should include an assessment of pain secondary to the inflammatory process and provision of treatment (e.g., applications of cold or heat unless contraindicated or use of mild analgesics or NSAID).

7 Pain in Special Populations

Recommendations

53. Clinicians should give special attention to the assessment and treatment of pain in special populations, including the very young and very old, cognitively impaired, known or suspected substance abusers, and non-English-speaking persons. (Panel Consensus)

54. Behavioral observation should be the primary assessment method for preverbal and nonverbal children and used as an adjunct to assessment for verbal children and cognitively impaired adults. (Panel Consensus)

55. Infants, especially nonventilated, should be closely monitored when they are administered opioids because opioid clearance is prolonged and the blood-brain barrier is more permeable, which increases their potential for opioid-induced sedation and respiratory depression. (A)

56. The elderly are more vulnerable to drug accumulation because of age-related changes in pharmacokinetics of analgesics; aggressive pain assessment and management are as necessary for them as for younger age groups. (A)

57. When new psychiatric symptoms occur in a patient with cancer, the possibility of uncontrolled pain should be considered. (Panel Consensus)

58. Uncontrolled pain, an important factor contributing to feelings of hopelessness, suicidal ideation, and requests for physician-assisted suicide or euthanasia, should be aggressively assessed and treated. (B)

59. Because patients with current substance abuse disorders are at risk for undertreatment of cancer pain, their care should be managed by clinicians knowledgeable in both pain management and substance abuse. (Panel Consensus)

60. Nonopioid analgesic modalities should not be substituted for opioid analgesics to treat severe pain in the suspected or known substance abuser. (Panel Consensus)

61. When assessing pain or developing a pain treatment plan, health care clinicians should be aware of the unique needs and circumstances of patients from various ethnic and cultural backgrounds. (Panel Consensus)

62. **Because patients with HIV positive/AIDS often have pain problems similar to those of patients with cancer, recommendations for pain assessment and management in this guideline are generally applicable for pain in these patients. (B)**

Pain in Neonates, Children, and Adolescents

Most children with cancer experience pain (McGrath, 1990b), which, as does the progression of cancer in children, differs from that of adults. After diagnosis, the common childhood malignancies generally respond rapidly to treatment, and disease-related pain often remits. If the tumor recurs and is resistant to treatment, the disease progresses rapidly, resulting in early death (Miser, 1993).

Pain in children with cancer arises more often from the treatment than from the disease (Miser, Dothage, Wesley, et al., 1987). Aggressive multimodal treatment protocols for children have increased survival rates markedly for most types of cancer, but they often involve treatment toxicity that results in painful conditions, e.g., mucositis, peripheral neuropathy, and infection.

Children with cancer undergo procedures ranging from venipunctures to bone marrow aspirations and biopsies. Children with aggressive treatment protocols may have one or more venipunctures daily, lumbar punctures weekly, and bone marrow aspirations monthly. Unlike adults, infants and children do not provide consent for these procedures and often do not understand the reasons for them or realize their short duration. Although appropriate preparation and adequate analgesia are crucial for children undergoing procedures, often neither occurs or they occur in a haphazard fashion (Schechter, 1989).

The optimal treatment of a child's cancer-related pain requires an awareness of the many factors that shape that pain. Among these are the child's developmental level, emotional and cognitive state, personality traits, physical condition, and past experiences; the meaning of the pain for the child; the stage of the disease; the child's fears and concerns about illness and death; issues, attitudes, and reactions of the family; cultural background; and the environment (Hester, Foster, and Beyer, 1992). Clinicians should be aware that children with cancer experience many distressing symptoms such as pain, depression, anxiety, panic, pruritus, fatigue, nausea, constipation, insomnia, dyspnea, and the fear of abandonment and death.

Getting to know the child and having knowledge of developmental norms and behavioral competencies are important in the assessment and management of pain. Clinicians should tailor assessment and management strategies to the child's developmental level, personality style, and emotional and physical resources and to the context; **tailoring is particularly necessary for children with developmental delays, learning disabilities, emotional disturbances, and language barriers.**

Assessment is not only diagnostic but also therapeutic. Assessing the meaning of the pain to the child and the family, the effect of the pain on the activities of daily living and on mood, and the concurrent concerns and symptoms helps clinicians understand pain from the perspective of the child and the family. Asking about pain underscores the clinician's desire to ease pain and suffering and builds a therapeutic alliance with the child and family.

It is easier for clinicians to understand inherently subjective experiences, such as pain, anxiety, and despair, when the child can verbalize, but for some children, verbal communication is difficult or impossible. Therefore, the clinician should recognize the potential for pain and discomfort or suspect that the child is in pain even if the signs are not immediately apparent.

Assessment

Whether the child is at home, in a clinic or clinician's office, or at the hospital, assessment of pain should occur during the course of his or her illness. Critical to assessment is open communication about pain among the child, the family, and the health care team.

An initial pain history focuses on understanding pain from the child's and family's perspective. Central to communicating with the child about pain is determining the language the child uses for pain (e.g., hurt, owie, boo-boo) and how and to whom the child communicates pain. Other issues include past pain experiences, the child's response to pain, expectations related to pain, and preferences for assessing and treating pain (see Attachment B). Clinicians should integrate this background information into subsequent assessments and treatment plans for the child.

A routine assessment of pain is critical to ongoing management. The frequency of assessment should be tailored to the severity of the pain, the context, and the preferences of the child and family. Frequent assessments are necessary when pain is being poorly managed or is not responding to the current treatment. Documentation of pain ratings on a chart or flowsheet, located in a visible place such as at the bedside, provides easy access for providers. The use of a flowsheet reduces the possibility of redundant questioning which can be overwhelming for the child and family and may interfere with the child's coping skills.

Methods for Assessing Pain

Assessment of children's pain involves one or more of the following approaches: self-reports, proxy reports, observations, and physiologic measures. "Because physiologic indicators such as heart rate, respiratory rate, blood pressure, and diaphoresis alter with a variety of stress-arousal events, they should not be used as measures of pain in the absence of other pain assessment methods or clinical indicators" (McGrath, de Veber, and Hearn, 1985). A variety of assessment methods are available, but no one approach provides a complete picture of the pain experience. At least one method that is reliable, valid, and developmentally appropriate to the child should be used regularly for assessing pain. Because children with cancer may need assessment in settings other than hospitals (e.g., their homes), the methods should be affordable and easy for parents or other caregivers to use.

Self-Report. Self-report methods provide the most reliable and valid estimates of pain intensity and location. These methods are appropriate for children over the age of 4 who can verbalize (McGrath, 1990b). Rarely will children with cancer fabricate pain (Ross and Ross, 1988), but they may deny or underreport pain if they (1) fear that admission of pain will mean further painful procedures or treatments such as "a shot for pain"; (2) lack awareness that pain can be treated; (3) wish to protect parents from the reality of progressive disease; or (4) desire to please and placate others.

Self-report methods should be easy to administer with simple instructions for children. They should allow both verbal and nonverbal (e.g., pointing) responses. Often, children will not respond to questions verbally, especially if they are anxious or depressed or are experiencing severe pain.

Several self-report methods for pain intensity are available for use with children (see Attachment B). Although the psychometric adequacy of these methods for children with cancer has yet to be determined, reliability and validity estimates are available for other pain syndromes such as postoperative pain, procedural pain, and juvenile rheumatoid arthritis. Methods appropriate for children over the age of 4 years include the Oucher (Beyer, Villarruel, and Denyes, 1993) and the Poker Chip Tool (Hester, Foster, and Kristensen, et al., 1989). Some investigators have used cartoon faces as scales of measurement for young children with cancer who are undergoing procedures, but the construct being measured was not necessarily pain. One scale measures pain affect (McGrath, de Veber, and Hearn, 1985), whereas others measure intensity of pain, anxiety, or distress (Adams, 1990; LeBaron and Zeltzer, 1984). Children over the age of 7 years who understand the concepts of order and number may prefer a numerical rating scale (NRS) (McGrath and Unruh, 1987), a horizontal word graphic rating scale (Savedra, Tesler, Holzemer, et al., 1989 [updated 1992]), or a VAS (McGrath, 1990b). A large study that included children and adolescents reported that the VAS was the least preferred of five horizontal pain scales (Tesler, Savedra, Holzemer, et al., 1991).

To determine the location of pain, children can be asked either to point to their body or use a body map (i.e., an outline). Children over the age of 4 can use crayons or colored markers to locate pain on a body map (Eland, 1989; Savedra, Tesler, Holzemer, et al., 1989 [updated 1992])(see Attachment B). The precision of the location will increase with the child's age. Children who are suffering may regress; similarly, children who are developmentally delayed or learning disabled may need assessment tools developed for younger children. If a child is unable or unwilling to provide pain ratings, parents or health care professionals can provide proxy reports. Proxy ratings, however, are inexact.

Behavioral Observation. Behavioral observation is the primary assessment approach for preverbal and nonverbal children and is an adjunct to assessment for verbal children. Observations focus on vocalizations (e.g., crying, whining, or groaning), verbalizations, facial expressions, muscle tension and rigidity, ability to be consoled, guarding of body parts, temperament, activity, and general appearance. Adequate reliability and validity documentation is lacking for behavioral observations; consequently, most such observations offer only a second-best approximation of the child's experience, even though clinicians often attribute greater importance to nonverbal expression than to self-report (Craig, 1992). Changes in how a child looks and acts may indicate the onset of pain or its increase (Hester and Foster, 1990) and warrant further investigation and documentation.

Observations are problematic in that the stimulus for behaviors or changes is not always clear. For example, children cry in response to pain, as well as fear, loneliness, and overstimulation. Clinicians may misinterpret behaviors such as sleeping, watching television, and using humor as the absence of pain when, in fact, the child is attempting to control pain. Moreover, behavioral responses may be absent or attenuated when vocalizations or movements cause or increase pain. Infants may become apathetic after only a few days of continuing severe pain, and suffering experienced by older children and adolescents with cancer may blunt behaviors and affect. Other factors that inhibit behavioral responses include intubation, use of paralyzing agents or sedatives, extreme illness, weakness, or depression. Therefore, the use of behavioral observation to guide analgesia requires close attention to the context. If caretakers are not sure whether a behavior indicates pain and if there is reason to suspect the presence of pain, a trial of analgesics can be diagnostic as well as therapeutic.

Most of the scales developed for measuring behaviors address postoperative pain or pain associated with invasive procedures (e.g., LeBaron and Zeltzer, 1984). Given the nature of cancer-related pain, behavioral scales for the assessment of acute pain problems are unlikely to be sensitive in assessing the child with cancer pain. The Gustave-Roussy Child Pain Scale (Gauvain-Piquard, Rodary, Rezvani, et al., 1987) is the only observation tool developed for children with cancer pain.

Pain Management

Pain is managed within a therapeutic alliance among the child, his or her parent(s), nurses, physicians, and other health care professionals. The beliefs and preferences of the child and family should be elicited, respected, and carefully considered. At the same time, the primary obligation of the health care professional is to ensure safe and competent care. The presence of divergent beliefs and goals among members of the team can interfere with effective pain and symptom management, but these can often be resolved through discussion and negotiation.

Medical Interventions. Medical interventions include analgesics, adjuvant agents (e.g., corticosteroids, tricyclic antidepressants, stimulants), palliative chemotherapy, radiation therapy, regional analgesia, and neurosurgical approaches. In most cases, analgesics—either alone or supplemented with chemotherapeutic agents, radiation therapy, and adjuvants—provide adequate pain relief. Regional analgesia is occasionally helpful.

Analgesics and Adjuvants. Health care professionals treating children often use medications that have not been specifically tested in children and that are thus not specifically indicated for pediatric use. This situation exists because children as a group are therapeutic "orphans"; the small number of children needing certain medications does not provide incentive for widescale testing. The administration of analgesics to children should follow the WHO's ladder approach (see Chapter 3). Usual doses for children are listed in Tables 8 and 10.

Acetaminophen and NSAIDs. Acetamenophen is a useful and relatively safe analgesic that provides effective relief of mild pain and enhances opioid effectiveness (Tobias, 1992). The rectal route is available for children who cannot take medication orally; however, children do not like this route and may refuse to take the medication. Rectal administration is contraindicated for children who are neutropenic or thrombocytopenic and for those with mucositis. These contraindications and the irregular absorption of the rectal route limit its usefulness in treating severe pain (Miser and Miser, 1989).

Because children with cancer are often thrombocytopenic, NSAIDs frequently cannot be used. They do, however, provide excellent analgesia for the child who is not at risk for bleeding because of thrombocytopenia or a coagulopathy and who is not at unusual risk of gastritis or ulceration (e.g., from the concurrent use of corticosteroids). NSAIDs effects on inflammation can be salutary, especially in the presence of bone pain. Evidence suggests that NSAIDs such as choline magnesium trisalicylate and salsalate have little effect on platelet function in normal subjects not at risk for bleeding (Cronin, Edmiston, and Griffin, 1991). Even so, the use of these "platelet-sparing" NSAIDs in children at risk for bleeding is not recommended.

The administration of acetaminophen and NSAIDs varies according to the severity of the pain (Table 9). For very mild or intermittent pain, as-needed administration is appropriate. However, hospitalized children and their parents should be told to ask for the medication if pain occurs. An advocate may be appointed to assist the child and parents in requesting medications. For continuous or more severe pain, around-the-clock administration is necessary (Table 9).

Opioid analgesics. For moderate to severe pain, opioid analgesics are recommended. Some health care professionals are concerned about the potential for addiction in children, a risk that is rare in adult cancer patients (Kanner and Foley, 1981). Although studies of the risks in children are lacking, no known aspect of childhood development or physiology increases the risk of physiologic or psychological vulnerability to chemical dependence. Therefore, withholding opioids from children with cancer is unwarranted.

Route of administration. Whenever possible, opioids should be administered orally. Many are available in a liquid form or suspension; often, those that are not commercially available in this form can be pulverized (with the exception of controlled-release drugs) and administered in a small amount of liquid or soft food.

Parenteral administration is indicated when:

- The child cannot take medication by mouth, for reasons such as obstruction, nausea, vomiting, and mucositis.

- Absorption may be compromised (e.g., as a result of chemotherapy-induced obstipation).

- The pain is severe and requires timely management and a rapid titration to effect.

- Frequent and severe breakthrough or incident-related pain occurs.

- The oral route requires frequent administration of medication or large numbers of pills or liquid.

Even with severe pain, once the opioid dose requirement is ascertained, the route can be changed over a few days from the intravenous to the oral route by using equianalgesic conversions (Table 11).

When parenteral administration is required, the intravenous or subcutaneous route can be used (Miser, Moore, Greene, et al., 1986). Some children with cancer have implanted central catheters, which can be used; similarly, children who cannot take medication by mouth often have an intravenous catheter for the administration of fluids, chemotherapy, or antibiotics. Intramuscular injections should not be used, because "shots" are painful and frightening to children.

Transdermal fentanyl provides an alternative route for children with relatively constant pain who require larger doses of opioid analgesia. It is unsuitable for rapid-dose titration or for any patient with changing pain intensity. Currently available preparations do not permit the delivery of drug at dosage rates low enough for young children.

Schedule and dose. Severe pain is an emergency, requiring the rapid titration of analgesia to provide relief within a few hours. Rapid titration involves frequent assessments and dosage adjustments. For example, because the peak effect of intravenously administered morphine occurs about 15 minutes after administration, the patient whose dose requirement is unknown could be given 0.1 mg/kg of morphine and be assessed every 15 minutes, with additional increments of 0.05 mg/kg administered until relief is obtained.

Opioids can be administered by intermittent bolus injections, infusions, or infusions with "rescues." Unless the pain is truly intermittent and unpredictable, as-needed administration should not be used since delay between the request for medication and the administration results in poor pain management. In those isolated cases when as-needed administration is indicated and when "rescue" doses of medication are added to an infusion, the child needs an advocate (e.g., nurse, parent) to ensure prompt administration.

Intermittent bolus injections of morphine or its analgesic equivalent can be provided on an around-the-clock basis at a starting dose of about 0.1 mg/kg. Initial dose intervals are the same as those recommended for adults. Continuous infusion of morphine, at a starting dose of 0.02 to 0.04 mg/kg per hour for children over 6 months of age has been well studied in postoperative pain and described in cancer-related pain (Hendrickson, Myre, Johnson, et al., 1990; Miser, Moore, Greene, et al., 1986).

Continuous infusion avoids the extreme variations that may occur with intermittent intravenous doses and is indicated when intermittent doses:

■ Cause undue somnolence at the time of peak effect.

■ Provide inadequate analgesia at the usual starting doses.

■ Must be administered more frequently than every 2 to 3 hours to provide adequate analgesia.

Children receiving a continuous infusion should be offered "rescue" doses for breakthrough or poorly controlled pain regularly on the basis of their level of pain and the duration of the effect of the prescribed opioid.

Because of wide variability in opioid dose requirements (Nahata, Miser, Miser, et al., 1984), pain and side effects should be assessed frequently, with the dose and interval adjusted for optimal relief. Many children require large doses of opioids; the process for dose increase and titration to effect is the same as in adults (see Chapter 3). To titrate to effect when a continuous infusion with rescue doses is used, the total amount of opioid administered (including rescue doses) is calculated for a specific time period, usually 8 or 12 hours. This amount is then added to the total amount of opioid to be infused over the next 8- or 12-hour period. Because four or five half-lives are required to reach a new steady state, increasing the infusion when pain is poorly managed will not by itself provide adequate, immediate relief. In fact, it could result in the administration of an unnecessarily large dose as soon as the infusion reaches a new steady state.

Agent. Morphine is the preferred starting agent for severe pain. Codeine and oxycodone can be used for moderate pain, although morphine and hydromorphone may be better tolerated by some children. Opioids such as hydromorphone, methadone (Miser and Miser, 1986), and fentanyl may be preferable when side effects are not easily controlled. Methadone use requires careful titration and appreciation of the potential for delayed somnolence because of its long half-life. Meperidine should be used only in exceptional circumstances such as hypersensitivity to morphine and hydromorphone and when a single dose (e.g., for a procedure) or use for fewer than 2 days is anticipated.

Patient-controlled analgesia (PCA). PCA provides safe and effective analgesia in children old enough to understand the relationship among a stimulus (pain), a behavior (pushing the button), and a delayed response (pain relief). Most children over the age of 7 understand this concept, and sometimes even younger children can learn to use PCA, but some may not have the cognitive or emotional resources to use it. Only one postoperative pain study has focused on the effectiveness of PCA with and without a basal infusion in contrast to the effectiveness of intramuscular morphine (Berde, Lehn, Yee, et al., 1991). One study addressed the efficacy of PCA for adolescents (age 18 or older) with cancer in treating mucositis after bone marrow transplantation (Hill, Chapman, Kornell, et al., 1990). Patient-controlled dose and basal infusion have not been explored systematically in children with cancer.

Monitoring. Regular assessment of a patient's vital signs and level of consciousness is necessary when parenteral opioids are used. Because of variable clinical situations and goals of treatment in children with cancer-related pain, professional judgment should be used to determine the presence, type, and frequency of monitoring. Because of wide interindividual and intraindividual variations in response, a child may have an adverse reaction, despite the most careful titration of doses and intervals.

Side effects. Young children may have difficulty communicating subjective symptoms like pruritus, nausea, constipation, and dysphoria; the preverbal child may show only generalized discomfort. If an infant or preverbal child becomes increasingly restless or irritable, despite an increased opioid dose, it is important to consider treatment of presumed side effects or a change to an alternative opioid. The pharmacologic approach to managing side effects in children is similar to that in adults. However, the assessment of side effects and pain relief should occur simultaneously.

One of the most feared side effects of opioid use is respiratory depression. In the dying patient, it may be due to the disease and not necessarily to the effects of opioids. In the patient who is not dying, naloxone may be indicated. If naloxone is used, it should be titrated incrementally (see Chapter 3) until the patient resumes adequate respiratory effort. The initial dose of naloxone in the child is about 0.5 to 2 μg/kg, with the dose repeated about every minute. Physical stimulation, oxygen administration, and support of respiration can be used while titrating the naloxone to effect.

Adjuvants. Tricyclic antidepressants can be used as described for adults in Chapter 3. In general, the starting dose should be low, (e.g., about 0.2 mg/kg of amitriptyline), and then increased to about 1 to 2 mg/kg daily. Tricyclic antidepressants should be used with care in children who have received large doses of cardiotoxic anthracyclines. A baseline electrocardiogram may be useful but is not required.

Stimulants such as dextroamphetamine and methylphenidate can also be used for children, with the goal being to provide additional analgesia and increased quality of awake time. The starting dose for both stimulants, 0.05 mg/kg, is gradually increased to effect with an upper limit of roughly 0.25 mg/kg per dose. Stimulants are given at times of desired wakefulness, such as morning and midday.

Analgesics for Neonates and Young Infants. Acetaminophen can be safely administered to neonates and infants without concern for hepatotoxicity when given for short courses at the recommended doses (Berde, 1991). Acetaminophen can be given to augment analgesia.

The use of opioids in young infants requires special consideration and expertise. Young infants, especially premature babies or those who have neurologic abnormalities or pulmonary disease, are susceptible to apnea and respiratory depression when systemic opioids are used (Purcell-Jones, Dormon, and Sumner, 1987). The infant's metabolism is altered so that the elimination half-life is longer and the blood-brain barrier is more permeable (Collins, Koren, Crean, et al., 1985; Lynn and Slattery, 1987). Both factors result in young infants having higher in-brain concentrations of opioids for a given dose than do mature infants or adults. **Intensive monitoring is reasonable up to about 1 year of age for nonventilated infants who are receiving opioids because extreme sedation and decreased respiratory effort may be difficult to assess.** Institutions where neonates and infants are treated for cancer should train personnel in the effective and safe administration of analgesia and provide appropriate technologies for monitoring.

Some evidence suggests that the clearance of opioids increases rapidly over the first few weeks of life and approaches adult levels by the time the infant is 1 to 2 months old (Hertzka, Gauntlett, Fisher, et al., 1989; Koren, Butt, Chinyanga, et al., 1985). Because available data are based on small numbers of infants, many practitioners reduce the initial dose and use intensive monitoring for infants up to 6 months of age; this age is arbitrary and represents a cautious interpretation of the literature.

Although further research is necessary, apnea and respiratory depression appear to be dose related (Koren, Butt, Chinyanga, et al., 1985). For nonventilated infants under 6 months of age, the initial opioid dose, calculated in milligrams per kilogram, should be about one-fourth to one-third of the dose recommended for older infants and children. For example, 0.03 mg/kg of morphine could be used instead of the traditional 0.1 mg/kg. Careful assessment is necessary so that the optimal dose and interval of administration can be determined from clinical parameters (e.g., when pain occurs and whether the infant appeared comfortable). Many infants have inadequate pain relief after the initial small dose and require upward titration, sometimes to doses equivalent to those used for older children. Continuous infusions can be used as long as the infusion begins with a conservative starting dose, which is then titrated upward until pain is relieved.

Aggressive monitoring, when necessary, should include frequent assessments and close observation of heart and respiratory rates, respiratory effort, blood pressure, and level of alertness as determined by responsiveness to stimuli. Frequent or continuous assessment of arterial oxygen saturation with pulse oximetry is a valuable adjunct to clinical observation. Because of delayed absorption, opioid levels in serum may increase many hours after a one-time intramuscular or subcutaneous dose in infants who are opioid naive; monitoring, therefore, should be continued for 12 hours after an opioid dose (Koehntop, Rodman, Brundage, et al., 1986).

Epidural Analgesia. The use of epidural analgesia is appropriate when systemically administered oral or parenteral analgesics do not achieve adequate pain relief without unacceptable sedation, respiratory depression, or other side effects. Epidural analgesia is now widely used for infants and children with postoperative pain. The hemodynamic and respiratory effects of major regional analgesia in infants with postoperative pain appear minimal (Meignier, Souron, and Le Neel, 1983). Systematic studies on epidural analgesia for children with cancer are unavailable, but experience in a few pediatric centers suggests that some children can be made comfortable with epidural or subarachnoid infusions of opioids and local anesthetics. For pediatric epidural infusion rates, the maximal recommended local anesthetic rates, per hour, are roughly 0.4 mg/kg for bupivacaine and 2 mg/kg for lidocaine. Epidural infusions that exceed those recommended rates may lead to convulsions (Berde, 1992). Epidural morphine has been used successfully even for young infants with cancer (Berde, Fischel, Filardi, et al., 1989). The proper use of infusions or intermittent doses of peridural opioids or local anesthetics requires expertise and close monitoring.

Nonpharmacologic Methods

Although little research has focused on the use of cognitive-behavioral methods for children with cancer, they have a potentially important role in relieving pain, and the methods used by adults can be adapted for children. For example, distraction techniques might involve reading or telling a favorite story, talking about the story's characters, or playing video games. Preparation for painful events could involve the use of a puppet, a favorite cartoon character, or an animal. Stuffed animals with inserted audiotapes of stories or music may help to induce a state of relaxation. Something familiar to the child may facilitate participation in these nonpharmacologic strategies.

When a child is in pain, the presence of a parent is usually helpful. Other methods of psychological support include holding someone's hand, a stuffed toy, or favorite blanket; asking questions; using distraction; sleeping and resting; relaxing or using imagery; changing positions; and engaging in humor; these seemingly simple interventions can have powerful effects. Facilitating the child's usual strategies for decreasing pain is important. Although not well researched in child populations, measures such as physical therapy, TENS (Eland, 1989), splinting a painful extremity, positioning, the application of heat or ice, and massage may help relieve pain (see Chapter 4).

Assessing the Adequacy of
Pain Management Strategies_____

The most important consideration in the management of pain in children with cancer is the provision of a child-centered environment and attitude. Health care professionals should understand and consider developmental issues and problems that affect the integrity and structure of the family. Child-centered cancer care provides the necessary items and services to support the child and the family emotionally, socially, and spiritually throughout the treatment process. In such an environment, pain and suffering are continually assessed, and appropriate supportive measures are introduced. Otherwise, the treatment of pain with analgesics and other agents will often be inadequate.

Optimal assessment and treatment require a knowledge of children's development, behavior, and physiology. Because children are less likely than adults to talk about pain, the responsibility to inquire about pain rests with the health care professional (Table 22). Some children will have pain that is particularly difficult to manage. In these situations, consultation with specialists in children's pain is recommended.

Elderly Patients

Elderly patients are often undertreated for cancer pain. Attitudes of health care professionals, the public, and patients toward pain can impede appropriate care; because many people consider acute and chronic pain to be a part of normal aging. In some instances, pain is not assessed because elderly patients, who may be confused, have difficulty communicating their pain to health professionals. In other instances, clinicians have mistaken beliefs about decreased pain sensitivity and heightened pain tolerance in the elderly. Frequently, the elderly are given nonopioids or weak doses of medications because their care providers mistakenly believe that they cannot tolerate opioid agents.

The elderly should be considered an at-risk group for the undertreatment of cancer pain because of inappropriate beliefs about their pain sensitivity, pain tolerance, and ability to use opioids. Elderly patients, like other adults, require aggressive pain assessment and management.

Pain management in the elderly presents several challenges, including the discrepancy between the high prevalence of pain in the elderly and the limited attention to this group in the research literature and in medical and nursing texts (Ferrell, 1991). Of all reports about pain published annually, fewer than 1 percent focus on pain experience or syndromes in the elderly (Melding, 1991). Current

Table 22. Checklist for assessing adequacy of pain management in children

---

Pharmacologic strategies

Have the child and parent(s) been asked about their previous experiences with pain and their preferences for use of analgesics?

Does the child or parent(s) have reservations about the use of opioids for pain treatment?

Is the child being adequately assessed at appropriate intervals?

Are analgesics ordered for prevention and relief of pain?

Is the analgesic strong enough for the pain expected or the pain being experienced?

Is the timing of drug administration appropriate for the pain expected or experienced?

Is the route of administration appropriate for the child?

Is the child adequately monitored for the occurrence of side effects?

Are side effects appropriately managed?

Has the analgesic regimen provided adequate comfort and satisfaction from the perspective of the child or parent(s)?

Nonpharmacologic strategies

Have the child and parent(s) been asked about their experience with and preferences for a given strategy?

Is the strategy appropriate for the child's developmental level, condition, and type of pain?

Is the timing of the strategy sufficient to optimize its effects?

Is the strategy adequately effective in preventing or alleviating the child's pain?

Are the child and parent(s) satisfied with the strategy for prevention or relief of pain?

Are the treatable sources of emotional distress for the child being addressed?

---

pharmacologic research is often limited to single-dose studies in young or middle-aged adults and does not assess the complications and side effects of medications in the elderly. Elderly patients who participate in pain clinics or studies are likely to be the mobile elderly. Furthermore, elderly patients are often excluded from rehabilitation programs and aggressive treatment of pain (Middaugh, Levin, Kee, et al., 1988; Sorkin, Rudy, Hanlon, et al., 1990).

In spite of the lack of research, there is evidence that the elderly experience more pain than younger people. It has been estimated that the prevalence of pain in those older than 60 years of age (250 per 1,000) is double that in those younger than 60 (125 per 1,000) (Crook, Rideout, and Browne, 1984). Among the institutionalized elderly, the prevalence of pain may be over 70 percent (Ferrell, Ferrell, and Osterweil, 1990). Elderly patients with cancer often have other chronic diseases, more than one source of pain, and complex medication regimens that place them at increased risk for drug-drug as well as drug-disease interactions.

Cognitive impairment, delirium (common among the acutely ill elderly), and dementia (which occurs in as many as 50 percent of the institutionalized elderly) pose serious barriers to pain assessment (Kane, Ouslander, and Abrass, 1989). Psychometric properties of pain assessment instruments, such as VAS, verbal descriptor, and numerical scales, have not been established in this population. Moreover, a high prevalence of visual, hearing, and motor impairments in the elderly impede the use of these tools. Research on the nursing home population shows that many patients with mild to moderate cognitive impairment are able to report pain reliably at the moment or when prompted, although their pain recall may be less reliable. **These findings suggest that this population may require more frequent pain assessment than patients who are not cognitively impaired** (Ferrell, in press).

Nonopioid analgesics, including acetaminophen and other NSAIDs, are helpful adjuncts to opioids for cancer-related pain. The risk for gastric and renal toxicity from NSAIDs is increased among elderly patients, however, and unusual drug reactions including cognitive impairment, constipation, and headache are also more common (Roth, 1989). Factors that may contribute to altered side effects in the elderly include multiple medical diagnoses, multiple drug interactions, and altered pharmacokinetics. If gastric ulceration is a concern, NSAIDs with lower gastric toxicity (e.g., choline magnesium trisalicylate) should be chosen. The coadministration of misoprostol should also be considered as a way to protect the gastric mucosa.

Opioids are effective for the management of cancer pain in most elderly patients. In the elderly, Cheyne-Stokes respiratory patterns are not unusual during sleep and need not prompt the discontinuation of opioid analgesia. Elderly people tend to be more sensitive to the analgesic effects of opioids, experiencing higher peak effect and longer duration of pain relief (Kaiko, 1980). The elderly, especially those who are opioid naive, also tend to be more sensitive to sedation and respiratory depression, probably as a result of alterations in metabolism and in the distribution and excretion of the drugs. For this reason, the prolonged use of longer acting drugs such as methadone requires caution (Ferrell, 1991).

Elderly people in general have increased fat-to-lean body mass ratios and reduced glomerular filtration rates. Opioids produce cognitive and neuropsychiatric dysfunction through poorly defined mechanisms that in part include the accumulation of biologically active metabolites such as morphine-6-glucuronide or normeperidine

(Melzack, 1990). Opioid dosage titration should take into account not only analgesic effects but also side effects that extend beyond cognitive impairment. Such side effects may include urinary retention (a threat in elderly males with prostatic hyperplasia), constipation and intestinal obstruction, or respiratory depression.

Local anesthetic infusions, including lidocaine or opioids, may result in cognitive impairment if significant drug levels in the blood are reached. Orthostatic hypotension and clumsiness may result from tricyclic antidepressant administration and other medications used for pain management and concurrent medical illnesses. Precautions, such as assistance during ambulation, should be taken to prevent falls and fractures.

PCA was shown to be safe and effective for postoperative pain relief among some elderly patients (Egbert, Parks, Short, et al., 1990). PCA has not been extensively studied for long-term use in the elderly with cancer-related pain. The use of any "high-tech" pain treatment such as PCA or intraspinal analgesia should be titrated and monitored especially closely because of the elderly patient's increased sensitivity to drug effects (Ferrell, Cronin Nash, and Warfield, 1992).

Patients With Psychiatric Problems Associated With Cancer Pain

Although patients with cancer and cancer-related pain commonly experience troublesome negative psychological consequences (Chapter 1), some patients require treatment beyond that provided by the patient's usual health care team. Three cancer centers (Derogatis, Morrow, Fetting, et al., 1983) reported that 53 percent of the patients were adjusting to the stresses of cancer with no diagnosable psychiatric disorder but that the remainder had clinically apparent psychiatric disorders. This study also noted that patients with pain were more likely to develop a psychiatric disorder; 39 percent of patients with a psychiatric diagnosis reported significant pain, but only 19 percent of patients without a psychiatric diagnosis had significant pain.

The incidence of pain, depression, and delirium all increase with higher levels of physical debilitation and advanced illness (Burkberg, Penman, and Holland, 1984). Approximately 25 percent of all patients with cancer experience severe depressive symptoms, with the prevalence increasing to 77 percent in those with advanced illness (Burkberg, Penman, and Holland, 1984). Among patients with cancer, the prevalence of organic mental disorders (delirium) requiring psychiatric consultation has been found to range from 25 to 40 percent and to rise to as high as 85 percent during the terminal stages of illness (Massie, Holland, and Glass, 1983).

Psychiatric symptoms in patients with pain should be viewed initially as a possible consequence of uncontrolled pain. Mood as well as personality characteristics may be distorted by the presence of uncontrolled pain, and relief of pain may result in the disappearance of a perceived psychiatric disorder (i.e., anxiety or depression) (Ahles, Blanchard, and Ruckdeschel, 1983). The patient's mental status should be reassessed after pain has been controlled to determine if a psychiatric disorder is present. The management of specific disorders such as depression, delirium, and anxiety in patients with cancer has been reviewed in detail elsewhere (Breitbart and Holland, 1988; Holland and Rowland, 1989).

Depression in Patients With Cancer Pain_____

The somatic symptoms of depression (e.g., anorexia, insomnia, fatigue, and weight loss) are less reliable and lack specificity in the patient with cancer (Endicott, 1984). Of greater diagnostic value are the psychological symptoms of depression: dysphoric mood, hopelessness, worthlessness, guilt, and suicidal ideation (Massie and Holland, 1990). A history of familial depression or of previous depressive episodes makes this diagnosis more probable.

An evaluation of cancer treatment-related organic factors that can present as depression should accompany treatment. Such factors include corticosteroids (Stiefel, Breitbart, and Holland, 1989), chemotherapeutic agents (Adams, Quesada, and Gutterman, 1984), whole-brain radiation (DeAngelis, Delattre, and Posner, 1989), CNS metabolic-endocrine complications (Breitbart, 1989), and paraneoplastic syndromes (Patchell and Posner, 1989).

Depressed patients with cancer are usually treated with supportive psychotherapy, cognitive-behavioral techniques, and antidepressant medications (Massie and Holland, 1990). The efficacy of tricyclic and other antidepressants in cancer patients is well established (Popkin, Callies, and Mackenzie, 1985). Psychostimulants are most helpful in the treatment of depression in patients with advanced disease and in those for whom dysphoric mood is associated with severe psychomotor slowing and even mild cognitive impairment. Clinicians are referred to the guideline on treatment of depression for further information on this subject (Depression Guideline Panel, 1993a, 1993b).

A patient's use of meperidine while on a monoamine oxidase inhibitor (MAOI) is absolutely contraindicated because it can lead to hyperpyrexia and cardiovascular collapse. One should be extremely cautious when using any opioid analgesics in patients on MAOIs, because myoclonus and delirium have been reported (Breitbart and Holland, 1988). Sympathomimetic drugs and other less obvious MAOIs, such as the chemotherapeutic agent procarbazine, can cause

Table 23. Risk factors that predispose cancer patients to depressive disorders

Social isolation.

Recent losses.

A tendency to pessimism.

Socioeconomic pressures.

A history of mood disorders.

Alcohol or substance abuse.

Previous suicide attempt(s).

Poorly controlled pain.

Source: Depression Guideline Panel, 1993a.

a hypertensive crisis in patients taking an MAOI. If a patient has responded well to an MAOI for depression in the past, its continued use is warranted, but with caution.

Suicide and Cancer Pain

Few patients with cancer commit suicide, but poorly controlled pain places them at increased risk. Tables 23 and 24 list factors that predispose cancer patients to depression and increase risk of suicide.

Although fleeting or occasional thoughts of suicide probably occur commonly in those with advanced illness, persistent and intense suicide thinking is rare in the absence of depression or of uncontrolled physical symptoms such as pain (Breitbart, 1990a). Suicide is often held as an option by the patient to retain a sense of control. Fear of unacceptable pain was a major component of requests to physicians for assisted death (Helig, 1988) and is so important to patients with cancer that 69 percent reported that they would consider committing suicide if their pain was not adequately treated (Levin, Cleeland, and Dar, 1985). In another study, the majority of patients who committed suicide had severe pain that was inadequately controlled (Bolund, 1985). Clinicians in a pain clinic report seeing many patients who considered suicide who changed their minds once given adequate pain relief (Foley, 1991). For at-risk patients, clinicians should be aggressive in the use of analgesics and other appropriate drugs as well as

Table 24. Suicide risk factors in cancer patients with pain

Depression.

Poorly controlled pain.

Previous suicide attempt(s).

Family history of suicide.

Delirium.

Substance abuse.

Prior psychiatric diagnosis (depression).

Advanced disease.

Increasing age.

Disfiguring disease or surgery.

Poor social support.

Source: Depression Guideline Panel, 1993a.

crisis intervention-oriented psychotherapeutic approaches that mobilize the patient's support system.

Although it is appropriate to intervene when medical or psychiatric factors are clearly the driving force in a suicidal cancer patient, overly aggressive intervention may be less helpful in patients with advanced illness when comfort and symptom management are the primary concerns. As an alternative to suicide, the goal of intervention should be to establish rapport, to develop an alliance, and to provide effective management of symptoms.

Anxiety

Although the experience of anxiety is a normal response when people learn they have cancer or in the case of recurrence or treatment failure, patients who continue to experience high levels of anxiety for weeks or months should be referred to a psychiatrist, psychologist, psychiatric nurse, or psychiatric social worker for evaluation and possible treatment. Some patients with cancer have long-standing or chronic anxiety disorders, such as phobias and panic disorder, that can be exacerbated by the stressors of cancer illness or treatment. Claustrophobic patients may experience acute anxiety when confined in diagnostic scanning devices or radiotherapy treatment rooms (Brennan, Redd, Jacobsen, et al., 1988). Patients who experience such acute anxiety or exacerbations of chronic anxiety disorders may require the use of medications such as benzodiazepines or cognitive-behavioral therapies to help them tolerate procedures.

Delirium and Its Effects on Treating Pain

Cognitive failure (delirium), common in patients with advanced illness (Fleishman and Lesko, 1989), is an etiologically nonspecific, global, cerebral dysfunction, characterized by concurrent disturbances of level of consciousness, attention, thinking, perception, memory, psychomotor behavior, emotion, and the sleep-wake cycle. Disorientation, fluctuation, waxing and waning of the above symptoms, and acute or abrupt onset of such disturbances are other critical features of delirium. Delirium is reversible, even in advanced illness. Still, it may not be reversible in the last 24 to 48 hours of life, most likely because of irreversible processes such as multiple organ failure (Massie and Holland, 1990).

At times, it is difficult to differentiate delirium from dementia because they frequently share clinical features such as disorientation and impaired memory, thinking, and judgment. One difference is that the temporal onset of symptoms is more subacute or chronically progressive in dementia than in delirium. Occasionally, delirium is superimposed on an underlying dementia, such as in the case of an elderly patient, an AIDS patient, or a patient with a paraneoplastic syndrome.

Delirium can be due to the direct effects of cancer on the CNS, to indirect CNS effects of the disease or treatments (medications, electrolyte imbalance, failure of a vital organ or system, infection, vascular complications) and to preexisting cognitive impairment or dementia.

Medical and nursing staff sometimes conclude that a new symptom is psychologically based without first ruling out all possible organic causes. Given the many drugs that cancer patients require and the fragile state of their physiologic functioning, even routinely ordered hypnotics can be enough to precipitate delirium. Opioid analgesics, including levorphanol, morphine sulfate, methadone, and meperidine (Bruera, Macmillan, Hanson, et al., 1989), can cause confusional states, particularly in the elderly and terminally ill. Clinicians should correct those underlying causes of delirium (Adams, Fernandez, and Andersson, 1986; Fainsinger and Bruera, 1992; Fish, 1991; Lesko and Fleishman, 1991; Lipowski, 1987).

Substance Abusers

There is a low risk of iatrogenic addiction in patients with cancer (Kanner and Foley, 1981). For patients with cancer who are additionally diagnosed as substance abusers, the complex physiologic, behavioral, and psychological phenomena associated with drug addiction in no way exclude the ability to perceive painful stimuli. When opioids are required for pain management, the concurrence of substance abuse disorders and cancer produces a difficult and stressful situation for even the most experienced clinician. Nevertheless, certain principles can be followed to assure a careful and fair assessment of the pain complaint and to provide the best chance of achieving satisfactory pain relief in these circumstances (Portenoy and Payne, 1992). These principles are complementary to those discussed elsewhere in this guideline.

Tolerance and physical dependence are predictable consequences of chronic opioid use, but they do not equal addiction (Newman, 1983). Numerous clinical, epidemiologic, and pharmacologic studies now suggest that cancer patients may become tolerant and physically dependent on opioids if therapeutic doses are prescribed for several weeks. However, very few patients develop the loss of control and compulsive use patterns that characterizes addiction to opioids (and other prescribed or illicit substances) despite medical, social, legal, or emotional harm. This sort of behavior, more than tolerance and physical dependence, characterizes and defines addiction (Portenoy and Payne, 1992).

An adequate assessment of the cause of pain is essential to the optimal treatment of the opioid addict with cancer. As with other cancer populations, specific antitumor treatments are indicated as the single best method of pain relief. Frequently, however, adequate analgesia has to be established before diagnostic studies and medical or surgical treatments can proceed. The appropriate management of the medical condition often decreases the requirements for opioids. Optimal pain treatment is essential to preventing the syndrome of "pseudoaddiction" (Weissman and Haddox, 1989) because inadequate pain management will invariably produce the manipulative behavior that the clinician wants to avoid.

Although not clearly substantiated by prospective clinical studies, it is common practice to make distinctions among (1) addicts who are actively abusing opioids and illicit narcotics at the time of their treatment for acute pain, (2) former addicts who no longer abuse drugs, and (3) addicts in methadone maintenance (Fultz and Sonay, 1975). Patients actively abusing heroin or prescription opioids (and those on methadone maintenance) should be assumed to have some degree of pharmacologic tolerance, which will be reflected in a need for higher-than-usual starting doses and dosing intervals shorter than those generally recommended in the nonaddicted population. Furthermore, because patients who are actively abusing drugs often manifest psychological disorders that influence pain perception (e.g., anxiety and depression), the treatment of concomitant psychiatric disturbances is often necessary and usually requires the consultation of experienced psychiatric clinicians. Patients with cancer who have abused drugs in the past (but who are not current abusers) or who are participating in methadone maintenance programs may have a higher degree of opioid tolerance than the general population. Among these patients, it is useful to anticipate that significant anxiety may accompany the stress of medical illness and acute pain and be manifested in a reappearance of drug-abuse behaviors.

The use of opioid agonist-antagonist compounds in known or suspected active opioid addicts is absolutely contraindicated. Not only do these drugs have ceiling effects to their analgesic efficacy, and are therefore inappropriate for severe pain, but they may also precipitate withdrawal and increased pain in physically dependent patients. **Likewise, nonopioid analgesic modalities should not be substituted for opioid analgesics to treat severe pain in patients who are suspected or known abusers of illicit substances.** Tolerance to opioid analgesics decreases the duration of effective analgesia (Houde, 1979); therefore, "tolerant" patients require more frequent dosing than do nontolerant patients. For example, morphine, which has an average analgesic duration of 3 to 4 hours, may produce only 1 to 2 hours of pain relief in an opioid addict with a large degree of tolerance.

Paradoxically, PCAs are being used with increasing frequency when rapid titration of intravenously administered opioids is required in this population. Although it would seem that the administration of opioids could not be entrusted to an addicted individual, in fact, it has its advantages: With the appropriate prescription of doses, "lock-out" intervals, and instruction to the patient, this method of administration may reduce the confrontation and conflict inherent in clinician-administered analgesia. Opioid addicts may report a euphoric feeling or "high" coincident with an intravenous bolus injection of opioids, which presumably reinforces the need to self-administer drugs (Jaffe, 1985). Nevertheless, intravenous opioids can be used effectively (see below).

Appropriate PCA bolus doses and "lock-out" periods (i.e., the time that should elapse between the administration of one dose and the next) should be selected. The opioid addict may be easily underdosed and experience poor pain relief if the degree of the patient's tolerance is not accurately assessed. The commonly published "lock-out" times and starting bolus doses are inappropriate for most opioid addicts and indeed for many patients whose prior opioid experience is such that they manifest opioid tolerance; in fact, the typical published parameters apply to the postoperative population of relatively opioid-naive patients. The prolonged self-administration of morphine to cancer patients with acute recurrent pain caused by oral mucositis after bone marrow transplantation did not increase the risk for over-medication or addiction (Chapman and Hill, 1989), and compared with standard intravenous infusion, PCA decreased the requirements for morphine by 53 percent (Hill, Chapman, Kornell, et al., 1990).

Although those patients were not addicts, the data nevertheless support the argument that PCA of intravenous morphine for pain does not invariably lead to ever-escalating dose requests.

Patients who are maintained on methadone for the treatment of addiction may also be treated with this agent for pain, if it is administered frequently enough. In this setting, methadone is useful in that the patient's dose may be easily tapered back to the level of the maintenance dose after the painful episode has been treated. In reality, however, most methadone maintenance programs do not have the flexibility to change the rules for individual patients to allow increases in the daily methadone dose or to increase the dosing frequency beyond once or twice a day. Unfortunately, then, the treatment of pain with methadone in this manner usually has to take place outside of the typical maintenance program.

For acute focal pain syndromes, regional anesthetic approaches such as somatic and sympathetic nerve block should be considered, unless contraindicated. These approaches are generally unsafe in patients who are septic, who have coagulopathy, or who are acutely confused and uncooperative. Nonpharmacologic methods can be useful adjuncts in the treatment of pain in this population.

One common characteristic of patients who are actively abusing opioids is a failure to set limits on their drug-seeking behavior, even in the presence of liberal uses of opioids for pain management. The clinician should discuss expectations and define limits of acceptable and unacceptable behaviors with the patient. The use of drug infusion pumps with security locks (available on almost all PCA pumps) should prevent dose escalation beyond what the clinician prescribes. If oral opioid analgesics are being administered, patients should be told that their ingestion will be witnessed and that routine precautions, such as searching the room for hidden pills or signs of hoarding, will be taken.

In the outpatient setting, clearly stated, written rules should cover prescription renewals, the procedure to be followed with lost or stolen prescriptions or medications, and procedures to ensure that only one clinician is prescribing analgesic medications. Prescription theft or forgery should lead either to the patient's admission to the hospital for continuation of opioid therapy, if still required, or to withdrawal of the therapy and referral to an appropriate drug treatment program, if opioid therapy for pain is no longer required. The patient should be seen frequently—daily, if necessary—and a limited quantity of opioids should be prescribed. In some States, the prescription of opioids to a patient known to be a "habitual user" or "addict" must be reported to the State's regulatory agencies.

These general guidelines allow the clinician and the patient to establish behavioral expectations, which may be the only way to manage humanely. **Patients with pain and substance abuse disorders require interdisciplinary assessment and care.** These patients are generally not well managed by the traditional medical models of oncologic care, because the issues of pain management and substance abuse treatment together are almost always beyond the competence of a single clinician or clinical service and may often produce directly conflicting goals for treatment. On the one hand, for example, the traditional method of opioid addiction treatment is to detoxify the patient and provide pharmacologic and psychological therapies to maintain abstinence. On the other hand, in treating the addict with cancer-related pain, the avoidance of opioids is usually unacceptable, because there are few alternatives for effective pain treatment. However, the pain specialist usually has little ability or training to assess fully the behaviors manifested by addicts, particularly those actively abusing drugs. There is no obvious solution to this paradox, but clearly, clinical research is needed to develop a model for the care of the addict with pain that allows flexibility of traditional concepts of substance abuse and pain management and provides a mechanism that effectively integrates both disciplines.

Minority Populations

In general, minority patients are likely to receive less adequate cancer treatment (Blendon, Aiken, Freeman, et al., 1989; Freeman and Wasfie, 1989). Indexing the adequacy of cancer pain management by WHO standards, a recent multicenter study found that minority patients (African-Americans and Hispanics) with pain due to metastatic cancer were three times more likely to have inadequate pain treatment than those seen in nonminority settings (Cleeland, Gonin, Hatfield, et al., in press).

The barriers that limit pain control in nonminority patients are even more likely to impede the pain management of minority patients. Cultural and linguistic differences may impair adequate assessment. Less frequent followup care will also lead to less adequate identification and monitoring of pain. Health care providers may be more concerned about the potential addiction of minority patients who need opioid medications on a chronic basis, and many minority patients may be more reluctant to use analgesics they see as potentially addicting. Because of concerns about theft and violence, pharmacies in neighborhoods where minorities live may not stock opioid analgesics (Kanner and Portenoy, 1986). Minority patients are more often economically disadvantaged, leading to inadequate reimbursement for pain control. Patients and families may face the dilemma of choosing between paying for pain medications or paying for other necessities.

Patients from special populations, because of their behavior when they have pain, may also be perceived as needing less aggressive pain management. Health care professionals frequently comment that such patients seem to have less pain even when they have equally severe tissue damage, because pain in these patients is inadequately assessed, but patients from diverse cultural and linguistic backgrounds will rate their pain at a similar level of severity when given the appropriate pain rating scales (Cleeland, 1989a). Judging pain by just observing the behavior of the patient will lead to consistent underestimation of its severity (Grossman, Sheidler, Swedeen, et al., 1991). **Therefore, when developing a pain treatment plan, health care clinicians should be aware of the unique needs and circumstances of patients from various ethnic and cultural backgrounds.**

Pain in Patients With AIDS

Pain is a symptom commonly experienced by patients with HIV infection, even in the absence of an opportunistic cancer such as Kaposi's sarcoma (O'Neill and Sherrard, 1993). The principles of pain assessment and treatment in the patient with HIV positive/AIDS are not fundamentally different from those in the patient with cancer and should be followed for patients with HIV positive/AIDS.

The reported prevalence of pain in HIV-infected individuals varies depending on stage of disease, care setting, and study methods. Estimates of the prevalence of pain in HIV-infected individuals generally range from 40 to 60 percent with prevalence of pain increasing as disease progresses (Breitbart, Passik, Bronaugh, et al., 1991; Lebovits, Lefkowitz, McCarthy, et al., 1989; Schofferman and Brody, 1990; Singer, Zorilla, Fahy-Chandon, et al., 1993). Thirty-eight percent of ambulatory HIV-infected patients reported significant pain in a prospective study of current pain prevalence (Breitbart, Passik, Bronaugh, et al., 1991). Fifty percent of patients with AIDS reported pain, while 25 percent of those with earliest stages of HIV infection had pain. Patients had an average of pain from two or more sources at a time. A review of ambulatory HIV-infected men (Singer, Zorilla, Fahy-Chandon, et al., 1993) demonstrated that 28 percent of those who were asymptomatic seropositive, 55.6 percent of those with AIDS-related complex, and 80 percent of those with AIDS reported one or more painful symptoms over a 6-month period. A study of pain in hospitalized patients with AIDS revealed that over 50 percent of patients required treatment for pain with pain the presenting complaint in 30 percent (Lebovits, Lefkowitz, McCarthy, et al., 1989). Schofferman and Brody (1990) reported that 53 percent of patients with far-advanced AIDS cared for in a hospice setting had pain. The most common pain syndromes reported in studies to date include painful peripheral sensory neuropathy, pain from extensive Kaposi's sarcoma, headache, pharyngeal and abdominal pain, arthralgias and myalgias, and painful dermatologic conditions (Breitbart, Passik, Bronaugh, et al., 1991; Lebovits, Lefkowitz, McCarthy, et al., 1989; Schofferman and Brody, 1990; Singer, Zorilla, Fahy-Chandon, et al., 1993).

HIV-related peripheral neuropathy is often a painful condition, affecting up to 30 percent of people with AIDS (Cornblath and McArthur, 1988), and is characterized by a sensation of burning, numbness, or anesthesia in the affected extremity. Several antiviral drugs, such as didanosine or zalcitabine, chemotherapy agents used to treat Kaposi's sarcoma (vincristine), as well as phenytoin and isoniazid, can also cause painful peripheral neuropathy.

Reiter's syndrome, reactive arthritis, and polymyositis are painful conditions reported in early HIV infection (Kaye, 1989). Other painful rheumatologic manifestations of HIV infection include various forms of arthritis (painful articular syndrome, septic arthritis, psoriatic arthritis), vasculitis, Sjögren's syndrome, polymyositis, zidovudine (AZT) myopathy, and dermatomyositis (Espinoza, Aguilar, Berman, et al., 1989).

Conditions associated with chronic or intermittent pain include intestinal infections with *Mycobacterium avium-intracellulare* and cryptosporidium, which cause cramping and intermittent abdominal pain; hepatosplenomegaly, resulting in abdominal distention and pain; oral and esophageal candidiasis, causing pain while the patient is eating and swallowing; and severe spasticity associated with encephalopathy, which causes painful muscle spasms.

HIV-related conditions that cause acute pain in children include meningitis and sinusitis, which result in severe headaches; otitis media; shingles; cellulitis and abscesses; severe candida dermatitis; and dental caries.

The patient with HIV disease faces many stressors during the course of illness including dependency, disability, and fear of pain and painful death. Such concerns are universal; the level of psychological distress, however, is variable and depends on social support, individual coping capacities, personality, and medical factors, such as the extent or stage of illness. In a study of pain in ambulatory HIV-infected patients (Breitbart, 1993), depression was significantly correlated with the presence of pain. In addition to being significantly more distressed and depressed, those with pain (40 percent) were twice as likely to have suicidal ideation as those without pain (20 percent). HIV-infected patients with pain were more functionally impaired, were more depressed, were more likely to be unemployed or disabled, and reported less social support.

Children with HIV infection often come from multiproblem families (Boland, Mahan-Rudolph, and Evans, 1989). Many families have more than one infected member, and multiple losses from AIDS in one family are common. These issues affect how families deal with the disease and the pain it causes. Parental guilt, which often results in denial of the disease, can also cause denial of a child's pain and resistance to adequate pain management.

Fears of addiction and concerns regarding drug abuse affect both patient compliance and clinician management of opioid analgesics and often lead to the undermedication of HIV-infected patients in pain. Also problematic is the management of pain in the growing segment of HIV-infected people who are actively using illicit drugs.

The issue of drug abuse is also problematic in the pediatric HIV population. Many children with HIV infection live in families where intravenous drug abuse is or was a problem. Either they have parents who are actively using drugs or are recovered from drug abuse, or they live with extended family who have had experiences with their drug-abusing relatives. In these environments, questions arise about the safety of prescribing opioids for the child. Extended-family members are often anxious about the use of opioids for a child whose parent was a drug addict, fearing that the child will also become addicted. These fears and concerns should be anticipated and discussed, and explicit plans such as those discussed earlier should be put into place to minimize the risk of drug diversion.

The general management of pain in children with HIV is the same as that for children with cancer. The assessment of pain in HIV-infected children may be complicated by the frequency of encephalopathy and related developmental delays. It is often difficult to determine whether an encephalopathic infant or toddler who cannot talk is in pain. Observations of a child's response to a trial of pain medication may be the best means of assessing such a child's pain (see Chapter 6).

8 Monitoring the Quality of Pain Management

Recommendations

63. To assure optimal pain management, formal means should be developed and used within each institution for evaluating pain management practices and for obtaining patient feedback to gauge the adequacy of its control. The quality of pain management should be evaluated in all settings where patients with cancer receive care. (C)

64. The quality of cancer pain management should be evaluated at points of transition in the provision of services (e.g., from the hospital to the home) to determine that optimal pain management is achieved and maintained. (C)

65. For pain management to be effective, each practice setting should designate who will be responsible for pain management. (C)

66. Policy and standard procedures, which define the acceptable level of patient monitoring and appropriate roles and limits of practice for health care providers, should govern the use of specialized analgesic technologies. (C)

To ensure optimal pain management, formal means should be developed and used within each institution for evaluating cancer pain management practices (American Pain Society, Committee on Quality Assurance Standards, 1990; National Institutes of Health Consensus Development Conference, 1987) **and should include feedback regarding the adequacy of pain relief.** Optimal pain management requires the interaction of all members of the health care team including the patient. A formal process should be developed to evaluate the quality of pain management across all stages of the disease and across all practice settings.

Quality pain management begins with an affirmation by health care professionals that patients should have access to the best level of pain relief that can safely be provided. In any setting, the quality of pain control is influenced by the training, expertise, and experience of clinicians. Practice settings vary considerably in size, complexity, resources, and patient populations. In addition, the goals of pain management may differ depending on the cause of the pain and the stage of the disease. Different pain management programs are therefore suitable in different practice settings, but the responsibility for pain management should always be assigned to the clinicians most knowledgeable, experienced, interested, and available to respond to patients' needs quickly.

One aspect of pain management that should be considered when evaluating quality of care is the multiplicity of settings where cancer care is provided. Patients with cancer receive care in ambulatory care centers, clinicians' offices, hospitals, their own homes, nursing homes, and hospices. **Pain management should be evaluated at points of transition in the provision of services to ensure that optimal pain management is achieved and maintained.**

The key items to consider when developing a formal program to monitor the provision of pain relief are:

- Patients' satisfaction with pain management and its impact on their quality of life.

- Family satisfaction with pain management and its impact on their quality of life.

- The designation of who is responsible for pain management.

- The systematic assessment of cancer-related pain in all settings where patients receive care.

- The accuracy of diagnostic approaches for common cancer pain syndromes.

- The range and appropriateness of pain management options available within a particular practice setting.

- The effectiveness of pain management options utilized to prevent and treat pain.

- The prevalence and severity of side effects and complications associated with pain management.

- The quality of pain management across points of transition in the provision of services (American Pain Society, 1992; Miaskowski and Donovan, 1992; Miaskowski, Jacox, Hester, et al., 1992).

The implementation of this guideline requires collaboration across disciplines and among clinicians. Three elements are essential for interdisciplinary collaboration: A common purpose, diverse professional skills and contributions, and effective communication and coordination of services (Spross, 1989). The common purpose is the relief of the patient's pain. To meet this goal, the diverse and complementary skills and contributions of each health care professional should be recognized and used. At times, however, interpersonal issues of power, leadership, and conflict can hamper efforts to relieve pain. Competent leadership and attention to conflict resolution are vital for building teams and keeping them focused on their shared purpose.

The following elements will help ensure effective communication and collaboration:

■ Clarity among professionals about what they can and will contribute (e.g., who will coordinate pain management—the primary nurse and attending physician or a specialized pain control team? Can consultants write prescriptions or orders?).

■ Decision making that reflects the input and preferences of the patient and family, such as providing a number of pain control choices that include pharmacologic and nonpharmacologic options.

■ Contingency planning, including orders to avert or treat possible side effects; a range of analgesic doses to deal with varying pain intensity; ongoing followup of cancer-related pain problems; and clear directions about whom the patient or caregiver should notify if changes in the plan are required.

■ In institutional settings, regular interdisciplinary meetings of clinicians to maximize communication and information sharing and to ensure appropriate planning.

The following recommendations (adapted from American Pain Society, 1992) should be implemented in every practice setting where patients with cancer receive care:

1. ***Promise patients attentive care.*** Patients should be informed, orally and in writing, that effective pain management is an important part of their treatment, that talking about unrelieved pain is important, and that health care professionals will respond quickly to reports of pain. It should be made clear to patients and families, however, that the total absence of any discomfort is not always an achievable goal.

2. ***Assign responsibility for pain management*** to clinicians most knowledgeable, experienced, interested, and able to respond to patients' needs in a timely fashion.

3. ***Document the assessment of pain and its relief.*** An assessment of pain intensity and pain relief should be recorded, regularly reviewed by members of the health care team, and incorporated into the patient's permanent record. The intensity of pain should be assessed and documented regularly (depending on the severity of pain) and with each new report of pain. The degree of pain relief should be determined after each intervention, once a sufficient time has elapsed for the treatment to reach peak effect. A simple, valid measure of intensity and relief should be selected, and the patient and family should be instructed in the use of the tool. For children, age-appropriate measures should be used (see Chapters 2 and 7).

4. ***Define pain and relief levels to trigger a review.*** Each practice setting should identify values for rating pain intensity and pain relief that will elicit a review of the current pain therapy. The proposed modifications in treatment should be documented, and the effectiveness of the modified treatment should be reviewed subsequently. Cleeland, for example, has shown that when patients indicate a level of "5" or above on a scale from 0 to 10, the patient's ability to function is markedly affected (Cleeland, 1984).

5. ***Survey patient satisfaction.*** At regular intervals, as defined by the practice setting and the quality improvement committee (if available), each setting should assess a randomly selected sample of cancer patients who have pain. Patients should be asked to rate their current pain intensity, the worst pain intensity in the past 24 hours, the degree of relief obtained from interventions, side effects associated with pain management, satisfaction with relief, satisfaction with the responsiveness of clinicians, and the extent to which their preferences in pain management were taken into account.

6. ***Analgesic drug treatment should comply with two basic principles:***

■ Oral analgesics and other noninvasive routes of administration are used whenever possible and administered in accordance with the principles expressed in the WHO analgesic ladder.

■ Analgesics are titrated to maximally effective doses or the appearance of dose-limiting side effects before specialized invasive analgesic approaches are used.

7. ***Monitor use of specialized analgesic technologies.*** **The administration of intraspinal opioids, systemic or intraspinal PCA, continuous opioid infusion, local anesthetic infusion, and conscious or deep sedation should be governed by policy and standard procedures that define the acceptable level of patient monitoring and appropriate roles and limits of practice for all health care professionals involved.** The policy should include definitions of physician and nurse accountability, physician and nurse responsibility to the patient, and the role of the pharmacist.

8. ***Offer nonpharmacologic interventions.*** Physical modalities and cognitive- and behavior-based interventions can provide substantial pain relief. Such interventions generally should be used to supplement, not replace, pharmacologic interventions.

9. ***Monitor the efficacy of pain treatment.*** Periodically review pain treatment procedures using the practice setting's quality improvement mechanisms.

References

Abboud TK, Zhu J, Gangolly J, Longhitano M, Swart F, Makar A, Chu G, Cool M, Mantilla M, Kurtz N. Transnasal butorphanol: a new method for pain relief in post-cesarean section pain. Acta Anaesthesiol Scand 1991;35(1):14-8.

Abel EL. Opiates and sex. J Psychoactive Drugs 1984;16(3):205-16.

Abram SE (editor). Cancer Pain. Boston: Kluwer Academic Publishers; 1989.

Acute Pain Management Guideline Panel. Acute pain management: Operative or medical procedures and trauma. Clinical practice guideline. AHCPR Pub. No. 92-0032. Rockville, MD: Agency for Health Care Policy and Research, Public Health Service, US Department of Health and Human Services; 1992.

Acute Pain Management Guideline Panel. Acute Pain Management: Operative or Medical Procedures and Trauma: Technical Appendix. Rockville, MD: US Department of Health and Human Services, Public Health Service, Agency for Health Care Policy and Research; in press.

Ad Hoc Committee on Cancer Pain of the American Society of Clinical Oncology. Cancer Pain Assessment and Treatment Curriculum Guidelines. J Clin Oncol 1992;10(12):1976-82.

Adams F, Fernandez F, Andersson BS. Emergency pharmacotherapy of delirium in the critically ill cancer patient. Psychosomatics 1986 Jan;27 (1 Suppl):33-8.

Adams F, Quesada JR, Gutterman JU. Neuropsychiatric manifestations of human leukocyte interferon therapy in patients with cancer. JAMA 1984;252(7):938-41.

Adams J. A methodological study of pain assessment in Anglo and Hispanic children with cancer. In: Tyler DC, Krane EJ, editors. Pediatric pain. Vol. 15. Advances in pain research and therapy. New York: Raven Press, Ltd.; 1990. p. 43-51.

Adams JE, Lippert R, Hosobuchi Y. Commissural myelotomy. In: Schmidek HH, Sweet WH, editors. Operative neurosurgical techniques: indications, methods, and results. 2nd ed. Vol. 2. Philadelphia: WB Saunders Co.; 1988. p. 1185-9.

Ahles TA, Blanchard EB, Ruckdeschel JC. The multidimensional nature of cancer-related pain. Pain 1983;17(3):277-88.

Akerman B, Arwestrom E, Post C. Local anesthetics potentiate spinal morphine antinociception. Anesth Analg 1988;67:943-8.

Amano K, Kawamura H, Tanikawa T, Kawabatake H, Iseki H, Iwata Y, Taira T. Bilateral versus unilateral percutaneous high cervical cordotomy as a surgical method of pain relief. Acta Neurochir (Wien) 1991;52(suppl.):143-5.

American Academy of Pediatrics. Guidelines for the elective use of conscious sedation, deep sedation, and general anesthesia in pediatric patients. Pediatrics 1985;76(2):317-21.

American Academy of Pediatrics Committee on Drugs. Guidelines for monitoring and management of pediatric patients during and after sedation for diagnostic and therapeutic procedures. Pediatrics 1992;89(6):1110-5.

American Cancer Society. Cancer and the poor: a report to the nation. American Cancer Society 1989.

American Cancer Society. Cancer facts and figures—1994. Atlanta: American Cancer Society Inc; 1994. p. 1.

American Cancer Society. Questions and answers about pain control: a guide for people with cancer and their families. American Cancer Society and the National Cancer Institute; 1992. p. 76.

American Nurses Association. Position statement on the role of the registered nurse (RN) in the management of patients receiving IV conscious sedation for short-term therapeutic, diagnostic, or surgical procedures. Nov. 1991. Available from American Nurses Association, 600 Maryland Ave., SW Suite 100 W; Washington, DC 20024.

American Pain Society. Principles of analgesic use in the treatment of acute pain and chronic cancer pain: a concise guide to medical practice. Skokie, IL: American Pain Society; 1986 [updated 1989, 1992].

American Pain Society. Principles of analgesic use in the treatment of acute pain and chronic cancer pain: a concise guide to medical practice. Skokie, IL: American Pain Society; 1992.

American Pain Society. Committee of Quality Assurance Standards. American Pain Society quality assurance standards for relief of acute pain and cancer pain. In: Bond MR, Charlton JE, Woolf CJ, editors. Proceedings of the Sixth World Congress on Pain. New York: Elsevier Science Publications; 1991. p. 185-90.

American Pain Society, Committee on Quality Assurance Standards. Standards for monitoring quality of analgesic treatment of acute pain and cancer pain. Oncol Nurs Forum 1990;17:952-4.

Angarola R. National and international regulation of opioid drugs: purpose, structures, benefits and risks. J Pain Symptom Manage 1990;5(2 suppl.):S6-11.

Angarola RT, Wray SD. Legal impediments to cancer pain treatment. In: Hill CS, Fields WS, editors. Drug treatment of cancer pain in a drug-oriented society. Vol. 11. Advances in pain research and therapy. New York: Raven Press, Ltd.; 1989. p. 213-31.

Arbit E, Galicich JH, Burt M, Mallya K. Modified open thoracic rhizotomy for treatment of intractable chest wall pain of malignant etiology. Ann Thorac Surg 1989;48(6):820-3.

Arcangeli G, Micheli A, Arcangeli G, Giannarelli D, La Pasta O, Tollis A, Vitullo A, Ghera S, Benassi M. The responsiveness of bone metastases to radiotherapy: the effect of site, histology and radiation dose on pain relief. Radiother Oncol 1989;14(2):95-101.

Ascari E, Attardo-Parrinello G, Merlini G. Treatment of painful bone lesions and hypercalcemia. Eur J Haematol 1989;43 (suppl 51):135-9.

Attardo-Parrinello G, Merlini G, Pavesi F, Crema F, Fiorentini ML, Ascari E, van Holten-Verzantvoort AT, Zwinderman AH, Aaronson NK, Hermans J, van Emmerik B, van Dam FS, van den Bos B, Bijvoet OL, Cleton FJ. Effects of a new aminodiphosphonate (aminohydroxybutylidene diphosphonate) in patients with osteolytic lesions from metastases and myelomatosis. Comparison with dichloromethylene diphosphonate. Arch Intern Med 1987;147(9): 1629-33.

Avellanosa AM, West CR. Experience with transcutaneous electrical nerve stimulation for relief of intractable pain in cancer patients. J Med 1982;13(3):203-13.

Bach FW, Jensen TS, Kastrup J, Stigsby B., Dejgard A. The effect of intravenous lidocaine on nociceptive processing in diabetic neuropathy. Pain 1990;40(1):29-34.

Baker DG. The radiobiological basis for tissue reactions in the oral cavity following therapeutic x-irradiation. A review. Arch Otolaryngol 1982;108(1):21-4.

Barbour LA, McGuire DB, Kirchhoff KT. Nonanalgesic methods of pain control used by cancer outpatients. Oncol Nurs Forum 1986;13(6):56-60.

Bates T. A review of local radiotherapy in the treatment of bone metastases and cord compression. Int J Radiat Oncol Biol Phys 1992;23(1):217-21.

Bates T, Yarnold JR, Blitzer P, Nelson OS, Rubin P, Maher J. Bone metastasis consensus statement. Int J Radiat Oncol Biol Phys 1992;23(6):215-6.

Bauchner H, Waring C, Vinci R. Parental presence during procedures in an emergency room: results from 50 observations. Pediatrics 1991;87(4):544-8.

Bauer W. Electrical treatment of severe head and neck cancer pain. Arch Otolaryngol 1983;109(6):382-3.

Baumann TJ, Batenhorst RL, Graves DA, Foster TS, Bennett RL. Patient-controlled analgesia in the terminally ill cancer patient. Drug Intell Clin Pharm 1986;20(4):297-301.

Beaver WT, Feise G. Comparison of the analgesic effects of morphine, hydroxyzine, and their combination in patients with postoperative pain. In: Bonica JJ, Albe-Fessard DG, editors. Proceedings of the First World

Congress on Pain. Florence, Italy. Vol. 1. Advances in pain research and therapy. New York: Raven Press, Ltd.; 1976. p. 553-7.

Beaver WT, Wallenstein SL, Houde RW, Rogers A. A comparison of the analgesic effects of methotrimeprazine and morphine in patients with cancer. Clin Pharmacol Ther 1966;7(4):436-46.

Beck SL. The therapeutic use of music for cancer-related pain. Oncol Nurs Forum 1991;18(8):1327-37.

Behar M, Magora F, Olshwang D, Davidson JT. Epidural morphine in treatment of pain. Lancet 1979;1(8115):527-9.

Bellville JW, Dorey F, Capparell D, Knox V, Bauer RO. Analgesic effects of hydroxyzine compared to morphine in man. J Clin Pharmacol 1979;19(5-6):290-6.

Berde CB. Convulsions associated with pediatric regional anesthesia. Anesth Analg 1992;75(2):164-6.

Berde CB. The treatment of pain in children. In: Bond MR, Charlton JE, Woolf CJ, editors. Proceedings of the Seventh World Congress on Pain. New York: Elsevier Science Publishers; 1991. p.435-40.

Berde CB, Fischel N, Filardi JP, Coe CS, Grier HE, Bernstein SC. Caudal epidural morphine analgesia for an infant with advanced neuroblastoma: report of a case. Pain 1989;36(2):219-23.

Berde CB, Lehn BM, Yee JD, Sethna NF, Russo D. Patient-controlled analgesia in children and adolescents: a randomized, prospective comparison with intramuscular administration of morphine for postoperative analgesia. J Pediatr 1991;118(3):460-6.

Beyer JE, McGrath PJ, Berde CB. Discordance between self-report and behavioral pain measures in children aged 3-7 years after surgery. J Pain Symptom Manage 1990;5(6):350-6.

Beyer JE, Villarruel AM, Denyes M. The Oucher: The new user's manual and technical report. 1st ed. February 1993. [Available from Judith Beyer, RN, PhD, University of Colorado Health Sciences Center, Denver, CO 80262.]

Beyer JE, Wells N. Assessment of cancer pain in children. In: Patt RB, editor. Cancer pain. Philadelphia: JB Lippincott; 1993. p. 57-84.

Blendon RJ, Aiken LH, Freeman HE, Corey CR. Access to medical care for black and white Americans. A matter of continuing concern. JAMA 1989;261(2):278-81.

Blitzer PH. Reanalysis of the RTOG study of the palliation of symptomatic osseous metastasis. Cancer 1985;55(7):1468-72.

Boland M, Mahan-Rudolph P, Evans P. Special issues in the care of the child with HIV infection/AIDS. In: Pediatric hospice care: what helps. Los Angeles: Los Angeles Children's Hospital; 1989. p. 116-74. See Ch. 7.

Bolund C. Suicide and cancer: II. Medical and care factors in suicide by cancer patients in Sweden. 1973-1976. J Psychosoc Oncol 1985;3:17-30. See Ch. 7.

Bonica JJ. Cancer pain. In: Bonica JJ, editor. The management of pain. 2nd ed. Vol. 1. Philadelphia: Lea and Febiger; 1990. p.400-60.

Bonica JJ. Treatment of cancer pain: current status and future need. In: Fields HL, Dubner R, Cervero R, editors. Proceedings of the Fourth World Congress on Pain; Seattle, Washington, Aug 31-Sept 5, 1984. Vol. 9, Advances in pain research and therapy. New York: Raven Press, Ltd.; 1985. p. 589-616.

Bonica JJ, Buckley FP, Moricca G, Murphy TM. Neurolytic blockade and hypophysectomy. In: Bonica JJ, editor. The management of pain. 2nd ed. Vol. 1. Philadelphia: Lea and Febiger; 1990. p. 1980-2039.

Botney M, Fields HL. Amitriptyline potentiates morphine analgesia by a direct action on the central nervous system. Ann Neurol 1983;13(2):160-4.

Brand F, Smith R, Grand T. Effect of economic barriers to medical care on patients' noncompliance. Public Health Rep 1977;92:72-8.

Breitbart W. Cancer pain and suicide. In: Foley KM, Bonica JJ, Ventafridda V, editors. Proceedings of the Second International Congress on Cancer Pain, Rye, New York, July 14-17, 1988. Vol. 16. Advances in pain research and therapy. New York: Raven Press, Ltd.; 1990a. p. 399-412.

Breitbart W. Endocrine-related psychiatric disorders. In: Holland JC, Rowland JH, editors. The handbook of psychooncology: psychological care of the patient with cancer. New York: Oxford University Press; 1989. p. 356-68.

Breitbart W. Psychiatric aspects of pain and HIV disease. Focus: A guide to AIDS research and counseling 1990b;5(9):1-3.

Breitbart W. Suicide risk and pain in cancer and AIDS patients. In: Chapman CR, Foley KM, editors. Current and emerging issues in cancer pain: research and practice. New York: Raven Press, Ltd.; 1993. p. 49-65.

Breitbart W, Holland JC. Psychiatric complications of cancer. In: Brain MC, Carbone PP, editors. Current therapy in hematology-oncology—3. Philadelphia: BC Decker Inc.; 1988. p. 268-74.

Breitbart W, Passik S, Bronaugh T, Zale C, Bluestine S, Gomez M, Galer B, Portenoy R. Pain in the ambulatory AIDS patient: prevalence and psychosocial correlates. Proceedings of the 38th Annual Meeting, Academy of Psychosomatic Medicine; October 17-20, 1991, Atlanta, GA. Chicago: Academy of Psychosomatic Medicine; 1991. p. 60.

Brennan SC, Redd WH, Jacobsen PB, Schorr O, Heelan RT, Sze GK, Krol G, Peters BE, Morrissey JK. Anxiety and panic during magnetic resonance scans. Lancet 1988;2(8609):512.

Bromage PR, Camporesi EM, Durant PAC, Nielsen CH. Rostral spread of epidural morphine. Anesthesiology 1982;56:431-6.

Brose WG, Cousins MJ. Subcutaneous lidocaine for treatment of neuropathic cancer pain. Pain 1991;45(2):145-8.

Brown DL, Bulley CK, Quiel EL. Neurolytic celiac plexus block for pancreatic cancer pain. Anesth Analg 1987;66(9):869-73.

Bruera E, Brenneis C, MacDonald RN. Continuous Sc infusion of narcotics for the treatment of cancer pain: an update. Cancer Treat Rep 1987;71(10):953-8.

Bruera E, Brenneis C, Paterson AH. Use of methylphenidate as an adjuvant to narcotic analgesics in patients with advanced cancer. J Pain Symptom Manage 1989;4(1):3-6.

Bruera E, Chadwick S, Brenneis C, Hanson J, MacDonald RN. Methylphenidate associated with narcotics for the treatment of cancer pain. Cancer Treat Rep 1987;71(1):67-70.

Bruera E, Macmillan K, Hanson J, MacDonald RN. The cognitive effects of the administration of narcotic analgesics in patients with cancer pain. Pain 1989;39(1):13-6.

Bruera E, Miller MJ, Macmillan K, Kuehn N. Neuropsychological effects of methylphenidate in patients receiving a continuous infusion of narcotics for cancer pain. Pain 1992;48(2):163-6.

Bruera E, Roca E, Cedaro L, Carraro S, Chacon R. Action of oral methylprednisolone in terminal cancer patients: a prospective randomized double-blind study. Cancer Treat Rep 1985;69(7-8):751-54.

Bruera E, Schoeller T, Montejo G. Organic hallucinosis in patients receiving high doses of opiates for cancer pain. Pain 1992;48(3):397-9.

Bullingham RES, McQuay HJ, Moore RA. Extradural and intrathecal narcotics. In: Atkinson RS, Hewer CL, editors. Vol. 14. Recent advances in anesthesia and analgesia. New York: Churchill Livingstone; 1982. p. 141-56.

Burkberg J, Penman D, Holland JC. Depression in hospitalized cancer patients. Psychosom Med 1984;46(3):199-212.

Byrne TN. Spinal cord compression from epidural metastases. N Engl J Med 1992;327(9):614-9.

Cain JM, Hammes B. Ethics and pain management: respecting patient wishes. J Pain Symptom Manage in press.

Campos RG. Soothing pain-elicited distress in infants with swaddling and pacifiers. Child Dev 1989;60(4):781-92.

Cassel EJ. The nature of suffering and the goals of medicine. N Engl J Med 1982;306(11):639-45.

Chapman CR, Hill HF. Prolonged morphine self-administration and addiction liability. Evaluation of two theories in a bone marrow transplant unit. Cancer 1989;63(8):1636-44.

Charlton JE. Current views on the use of nerve blocking in the relief of chronic pain. In: Swerdlow M, editor. The therapy of pain. 2nd edition. Lancaster: MTP Press, Ltd.; 1986. p. 133-64.

Chauvin M, Samii K, Schermann JM, Sandouk P, Bourdon R, Viars P. Plasma pharmacokinetics of morphine after i.m., extradural and intrathecal administration. Br J Anaesth 1982;54(8):843-7.

Choi CR, Ha YS, Ahn MS, Lee JS, Song JU. Intraventricular or epidural injection of morphine for severe pain. Neurochirurgia (Stuttg) 1989;32(6):180-3.

Citron ML, Johnston-Early A, Boyer M, Krasnow SH, Hood M, Cohen MH. Patient-controlled analgesia for severe cancer pain. Arch Intern Med 1986;146(4):734-6.

Cleeland CS. Barriers to the management of cancer pain. Oncology 1987;1(2 suppl.):19-26.

Cleeland CS. Management of cancer pain. Clin Cancer Briefs 1985;7(3):3-12.

Cleeland CS. Measurement of pain by subjective report. In: Chapman CR, Loeser JD, editors. Issues in pain measurement. Vol. 12. Advances in pain research and therapy. New York: Raven Press, Ltd.; 1989a. p. 391-404.

Cleeland CS. Pain control: public and physicians' attitudes. In: Hill CS Jr, Fields WS, editors. Drug treatment of cancer pain in a drug-oriented society. Vol. 11. Advances in pain research and therapy. New York: Raven Press, Ltd.; 1989b. p. 81-9.

Cleeland CS. The impact of pain on the patient with cancer. Cancer 1984;54:2635-41.

Cleeland CS, Cleeland LM, Dar R, Rinehardt LC. Factors influencing physician management of cancer pain. Cancer 1986;58(3):796-800.

Cleeland CS, Gonin R, Hatfield AK, Edmonson JH, Blum RH, Stewart JA, Pandya KJ. Pain and pain treatment in outpatients with metastatic cancer: the Eastern Cooperative Oncology Group's Outpatient Pain Study. N Engl J Med; in press.

Cleeland CS, Syrjala KL. How to assess cancer pain. In: Turk D, Melzack R, editors. Pain assessment. New York: Guilford Press; 1992. p. 360-87.

Cohn ML, Machado AF, Bier R, Cohn M. Piroxicam and doxepin—an alternative to narcotic analgesics in managing advanced cancer pain. West J Med 1988;148(3):303-6.

Collins C, Koren G, Crean P, Klein J, Roy WL, MacLeod SM. Fentanyl pharmacokinetics and hemodynamic effects in preterm infants during ligation of patent ductus arteriosus. Anesth Analg 1985;64(11):1078-80.

Controlled Substances Act, 21 U.S.C., sec 802. (West, 1981).

Cook PR, Campbell FN, Puddy BR. Pituitary alcohol injection for cancer pain. Anesthesia 1984;39(6):540-5.

Cornblath DR, McArthur JC. Predominantly sensory neuropathy in patients with AIDS and AIDS-related complex. Neurology 1988;38(5):794-6.

Cousins MJ. The spinal route of analgesia. Acta Anaesthesiol Belg 1988;39(3 suppl. 2):71-82.

Cousins MJ, Bridenbaugh PO, editors. Neural blockade in clinical anesthesia and management of pain. 2nd ed. Philadelphia: JB Lippincott Co.; 1987. p. 1171.

Cousins MJ, Mather LE. Intrathecal and epidural administration of opioids. Anesthesiology 1984;61:276-310.

Coyle N, Adelhardt J, Foley KM, Portenoy RK. Character of terminal illness in the advanced cancer patient: pain and other symptoms during the last four weeks of life. J Pain Symptom Manage 1990;5(2):83-93.

Craig KD. The facial expression of pain: better than a thousand words? APS Journal 1992;1(3):153-62.

Cronin C, Edmiston K, Griffin T. Hematologic safety of choline magnesium trisalicylate: a non-opioid analgesic. J Pain Symptom Manage 1991;6(3):158.

Crook J, Rideout E, Browne G. The prevalence of pain complaints in a general population. Pain 1984;18(3):299-314.

Dahl JL, Joranson DE, Engber D, Dosch J. The cancer pain problem: Wisconsin's response. A report on the Wisconsin Cancer Pain Initiative. J Pain Symptom Manage 1988;3(1):S1-20.

Danesh BJ, Saniabadi AR, Russell RI, Lowe GD. Therapeutic potential of choline magnesium trisalicylate as an alternative to aspirin for patients with bleeding tendencies. Scott Med J 1987;32(6):167-8.

Dar R, Beach CM, Barden PL, Cleeland CS. Cancer pain in the marital system: a study of patients and their spouses. J Pain Symptom Manage 1992;7(2):87-93.

Daut RL, Cleeland CS. The prevalence and severity of pain in cancer. Cancer 1982;50(9):1913-8.

Davis GC, Cortex C, Rubin BR. Pain management in the older adult with rheumatoid arthritis or osteoarthritis. Arthritis Care Res 1990;3(3):127-31.

Davis LE, Drachman DB. Myeloma neuropathy. Successful treatment of two patients and review of cases. Arch Neurol 1972;27(6):507-11.

Day RO, Furst DE, Graham GG, Champion GD. The clinical pharmacology of aspirin and the salicylates. In: Paulus HE, Furst DE, Dromgoole SH, editors. Anti-inflammatory agents, non-steroidal. Vol. 16. Drugs for rheumatic disease. New York: Churchill Livingstone; 1987. p. 227-64.

DeAngelis LM, Delattre JY, Posner JB. Radiation-induced dementia in patients cured of brain metastases. Neurology 1989;39(6):789-96.

Dejgard A, Petersen P, Kastrup J. Mexiletine for treatment of chronic painful diabetic neuropathy. Lancet 1988;1:9-11.

Delmas PD, Charhon S, Chapuy MC, Vignon E, Briancon D, Edouard C, Meunier PJ. Long-term effects of dichloromethylene diphosphonate (Cl$_2$MDP) on skeletal lesions in multiple myeloma. Metab Bone Dis Relat Res 1982;4(3):163-8.

Depression Guideline Panel. Depression in Primary Care: Vol. 1. Detection and Diagnosis. Clinical Practice Guideline. Number 5. Rockville, MD: US Department of Health and Human Services, Public Health Service, Agency for Health Care Policy and Research. AHCPR Pub. No. 93-0550; April 1993a.

Depression Guideline Panel. Depression in Primary Care: Vol. 2. Treatment of Major Depression. Clinical Practice Guideline. Number 5. Rockville, MD: US Department of Health and Human Services, Public Health Service, Agency for Health Care Policy and Research. AHCPR Pub. No. 93-0551; April 1993b.

Derogatis LR, Morrow GR, Fetting J, Penman D, Piasetsky S, Schmale AM, Henrichs M, Carnicke CL Jr. The prevalence of psychiatric disorders among cancer patients. JAMA 1983;249(6):751-7.

Donovan MI, Dillon P. Incidence and characteristics of pain in a sample of hospitalized cancer patients. Cancer Nurs 1987;10(2):85-92.

Dray A. Epidural opiates and urinary retention: new models provide new insights. Anesthesiology 1988;68(3):323-4.

Dreizen S. Oral complications of cancer therapies. Description and incidence of oral complications. NCI Monogr 1990;9:11-5.

Dunphy JE. Annual discourse—on caring for the patient with cancer. New Engl J Med 1976;295(6):313-19.

Du Pen SL, Peterson DG, Williams A, Bogosian AJ. Infection during chronic epidural catheterization: diagnosis and treatment. Anesthesiology 1990;73:905-9.

Du Pen SL, Ramsey D, Chin S. Chronic epidural morphine and preservative-induced injury. Anesthesiology 1987;67(6):987-8.

Du Pen SL, Williams AR. Management of patients receiving combined epidural morphine and bupivacaine for the treatment of cancer pain. J Pain Symptom Manage 1992;7(2):125-7.

Egbert AM, Parks LH, Short LM, Burnett ML. Randomized trial of postoperative patient-controlled analgesia vs intramuscular narcotics in frail elderly men. Arch Intern Med 1990;150(9):1897-903.

Eisenberg E, Carr D, Chalmers T. Neurolytic celiac plexus block for treatment of cancer pain: a meta-analysis. Submitted for publication.

Eland JM. The effectiveness of transcutaneous electrical nerve stimulation (TENS) with children experiencing cancer pain. In: Funk SG, Tornquist EM, Champagne MT, Copp LA, Wiese RA, editors. Key aspects of comfort: management of pain, fatigue, and nausea. New York: Springer Publishing Co.; 1989. p. 87-100.

Ellerton ML, Caty S, Ritchie JA. Helping young children master intrusive procedures through play. Child Health Care 1985 Spr;13(4):167-73.

Elliott K, Foley KM. Neurologic pain syndromes in patients with cancer. Neurol Clin 1989;7(2):333-60.

Ellison NM. Opioid analgesics: toxicities and their treatments. In: Patt RB, editor. Cancer pain. Philadelphia: JB Lippincott Co.; 1993. p. 185-94.

Elomaa I, Blomqvist C, Grohn P, Porkka L, Kairento AL, Selander K, Lamberg-Allardt C, Holmstrom T. Long-term controlled trial with diphosphonate in patients with osteolytic bone metastases. Lancet 1983;1(8317):146-9.

Endicott J. Measurement of depression in patients with cancer. Cancer 1984;53(10 suppl.):2243-9.

Epstein JB. Infection prevention in bone marrow transplantation and radiation patients. NCI Monogr 1990;9:73-85.

Espinoza LR, Aguilar JL, Berman A, Gutierrez F, Vascy FB, Germain BF. Rheumatic manifestations associated with human immunodeficiency virus infection. Arthritis Rheum 1989;32(12):1615-22.

Estes D, Kaplan K. Lack of platelet effect with the aspirin analog, salsalate. Arthritis Rheum 1980;23(11):1303-7.

Evans PJ, Lloyd JW, Jack TM. Cryoanalgesia for intractable perineal pain. J R Soc Med 1981;74(11):804-9.

Facing forward: A guide for cancer survivors. US Department of Health and Human Services, Public Health Service, National Institutes of Health, National Cancer Institute, July 1990. NIH Pub. No. 90-2424, p. 43.

Fainsinger R, Bruera E. Treatment of delirium in a terminally ill patient. J Pain Symptom Manage 1992;7(1):54-6.

Fairchild VM, Salerno LM, Wedding SL, Weinberg E. Physical therapy. In: Raj PP, editor. Practical management of pain: with special emphasis on physiology of pain syndromes and techniques of management. Chicago: Yearbook Medical Publishers; 1986. p. 839-52.

Fawzy FI, Cousins N, Fawzy NW, Kemeny ME, Elashoff R, Morton D. A structured psychiatric intervention for cancer patients. I. Changes over time in methods of coping and affective disturbance. Arch Gen Psychiatry 1990;47(8):720-5.

Ferrante FM, Ostheimer GW, Covino BG, editors. Patient-controlled analgesia. Boston: Blackwell Scientific Publications; 1990.

Ferrell BA. Assessment and management of pain in nursing homes. Ann Intern Med, (in press for Annals of Internal Med. 1994).

Ferrell BA. Pain management in elderly people. J Am Geriatr Soc 1991;39(1):64-73.

Ferrell BA, Ferrell BR, Osterweil D. Pain in the nursing home. J Am Geriatr Soc 1990;38(4):409-14.

Ferrell BR, Griffith H. Cost issues related to pain management. J Pain Symptom Manage in press.

Ferrell BR, Cohen MZ, Rhiner M, Rozek A. Pain as a metaphor for illness. Part II: Family caregivers' management of pain. Oncol Nurs Forum 1991;18(8):1315-21.

Ferrell BR, Cronin Nash C, Warfield C. The role of patient-controlled analgesia in the management of cancer pain. J Pain Symptom Manage 1992;7(3):149-54.

Ferrell BR, Rhiner M, Cohen MZ, Grant M. Pain as a metaphor for illness. Part I: Impact of cancer pain on family caregivers. Oncol Nurs Forum 1991;18(8):1303-9.

Ferrell BR, Rhiner M, Ferrell BA. Development and implementation of a pain education program. Cancer 1993;72(11 suppl.):3426-32.

Ferris FD, Kerr IG, Sone M, Marcuzzi M. Transdermal scopolamine use in the control of narcotic-induced nausea. J Pain Symptom Manage 1991;6(6):389-93.

Fields HL, Basbaum AI. Brainstem control of spinal pain-transmission neurons. Annu Rev Physiol 1978;40:217-48.

Fine PG. Nerve blocks, herpes zoster, and postherpetic neuralgia. In: Watson CPN, editor. Pain research and clinical management. Vol. 8. Herpes zoster and postherpetic neuralgia. New York: Elsevier Science Publishers; 1993. p. 173-83.

Fish DN. Treatment of delirium in the critically ill patient. Clin Pharm 1991;10(6):456-66.

Fishman B, Pasternak S, Wallenstein SL, Houde RW, Holland JC, Foley KM. The Memorial Pain Assessment Card: a valid instrument for the evaluation of cancer pain. Cancer 1987;60(5):1151-8.

Fleisch H, Russel RGG, Francis MD. Diphosphonates inhibit hydroxyapatite dissolution in vitro and bone resorption in tissue culture in vivo. Science 1969;165:1262-4.

Fleishman SB, Lesko LM. Delirium and dementia. In: Holland JC, Rowland JH, editors. The handbook of psychooncology: psychological care of the patient with cancer. New York: Oxford University Press; 1989. p. 342-55.

Foley KM. Brachial plexopathy in patients with breast cancer. In: Harris JR, Hellman S, Henderson IC, Kinne DW, editors. Breast diseases. Philadelphia: JB Lippincott Co.; 1987. p. 532-7.

Foley KM. Pain syndromes in patients with cancer. In: Bonica JJ, Ventafridda V, editors. International Symposium on Pain of Advanced Cancer; 1978; Venice. Vol. 2. Advances in pain research and therapy. New York: Raven Press, Ltd.; 1979. p. 59-75.

Foley KM. The treatment of cancer pain. N Engl J Med 1985a;313(2):84-95.

Foley KM. Overview of cancer pain and brachial and lumbosacral plexopathy. In: Management of cancer pain: syllabus of the postgraduate course, Memorial Sloan-Kettering Cancer Center, 1985 Nov 14-16. New York: Memorial Sloan-Kettering Cancer Center; 1985b. p. 25-50.

Foley KM. Changing concepts of tolerance to opioids: what the cancer patient has taught us. In: Chapman CR, Foley KM, editors. Current and emerging issues in cancer pain: research and practice. New York: Raven Press, Ltd.; 1993. p. 331-50.

Foley KM. The relationship of pain and symptom management to patient requests for physician-assisted suicide. J Pain Symptom Manage 1991;6(5):289-97.

Forrest WH Jr, Brown BW Jr, Brown CR, Defalque R, Gold M, Gordon HE, James KE, Katz J, Mahler DL, Schroff P, Teutsch G. Dextroamphetamine with morphine for the treatment of postoperative pain. N Engl J Med 1977;296(13):712-5.

Fowler-Kerry S. Adolescent oncology survivors' recollection of pain. In: Tyler DC, Krane EJ, editors. First International Pain Symposium, Seattle, Washington, July 1988. Pediatric pain. Vol. 15. Advances in pain research and therapy. New York: Raven Press, Ltd.; 1990. p. 365-72.

France RD. The future for antidepressants: treatment of pain. Psychopathology 1987;20(suppl. 1):99-113.

Fraser HM, Chapman V, Dickenson AH. Spinal local anaesthetic actions on afferent evoked responses and wind-up of nociceptive neurones in the rat spinal cord: combination with morphine produces marked potentiation of antinociception. Pain 1992;49:33-41.

Freeman HP, Wasfie TJ. Cancer of the breast in poor black women. Cancer 1989;63(12):2562-9.

French LA, Galicich JH. The use of steroids for control of cerebral edema. Clin Neurosurg 1964;10:212-23.

Fultz JM, Sonay EC. Guidelines for the management of hospitalized narcotic addicts. Ann Intern Med 1975;82(6):815-8.

Galasko CSB. Skeletal metastases and mammary cancer. Ann Roy Surg Engl 1972;50:2-28.

Galer BS, Coyle N, Pasternak GW, Portenoy RK. Individual variability in the response to different opioids: report of five cases. Pain 1992;49:87-91.

Gauvain-Piquard A, Rodary C, Rezvani A, Lemerle J. Pain in children aged 2-6 years: a new observational rating scale elaborated in a pediatric oncology unit—preliminary report. Pain 1987;31(2):177-88.

Gerbershagen HU. Neurolysis. Subarachnoid neurolytic blockade. Acta Anaesthesiol Belg 1981;32(1):44-57.

Gilbert RW, Kim JH, Posner JB. Epidural spinal cord compression from metastatic tumor: diagnosis and treatment. Ann Neurol 1978;3(1):40-51.

Gildenberg PL. Myelotomy and percutaneous cervical cordotomy for the treatment of cancer pain. Appl Neurophysiol 1984;47(4-6):208-15.

Giorgi C, Broggi G. Surgical treatment of glossopharyngeal neuralgia and pain from cancer of the nasopharynx. A 20-year experience. J Neurosurg 1984;61(5);952-5.

Glare P, Lickiss JN. Unrecognized constipation in patients with advanced cancer: a recipe for therapeutic disaster. J Pain Symptom Manage 1992;7(6):369-71.

Glazier HS. Potentiation of pain relief with hydroxyzine: a therapeutic myth? In: Thompson DF, editor. Therapeutic controversies. DICP Ann Pharmacother 1990;24:484-8.

Goisis A, Gorini M, Ratti R, Luliri P. Application of a WHO protocol on medical therapy for oncologic pain in an internal medicine hospital. Tumori 1989;75:470-2.

Gol A. Relief of pain by electrical stimulation of the septal area. J Neurol Sci 1967;5(1):115-20.

Gonzales GR, Payne R, Foley KM, Portenoy RK. Prevalence and character-istics of brachial plexopathy in a large cancer center: a retrospective study. Third Annual Bristol-Meyers Pain Research Symposium, Seattle; 1992.

Gracely RH, Wolskee PJ. Semantic functional measurement of pain: integrat-ing perception and language. Pain 1983;15(4):389-98.

Graffam S, Johnson A. A comparison of two relaxation strategies for the relief of pain and its distress. J Pain Symptom Manage 1987;2(4):229-31.

Greenberg HS, Deck MD, Vikram B, Chu FC, Posner JB. Metastasis to the base of the skull: clinical findings in 43 patients. Neurology 1981;31(5):530-7.

Greenberg HS, Kim JH, Posner JB. Epidural spinal cord compression from metastatic tumor: results with a new treatment protocol. Ann Neurol 1980;8(4):361-6.

Greenwald HP, Bonica JJ, Bergner M. The prevalence of pain in four cancers. Cancer 1987;60(10):2563-9.

Grond S, Zech D, Schug SA, Lynch J, Lehmann KA. Validation of World Health Organization guidelines for cancer pain relief during the last days and hours of life. J Pain Symptom Manage 1991;6(7):411-22.

Grossman SA, Sheidler VR, Swedeen K, Mucenski J, Piantadosi S. Correlation of patient and caregiver ratings of cancer pain. J Pain Symptom Manage 1991;6(2):53-7.

Gybels J. The role of spinal cord stimulation in contemporary pain management: a commentary. APS Journal Summer 1993;2(2):100-2.

Gybels JM, Sweet WH. Neurosurgical treatment of persistent pain. New York: Karger; 1989.

Hagen NA, Foley KM, Cerbone DJ, Portenoy RK, Inturrisi CE. Chronic nausea and morphine-6-glucuronide. J Pain Symptom Manage 1991;6(3):125-8.

Hall EJ. Nine decades of radiobiology: is radiation therapy any better for it? Cancer 1993;71:3753-66.

Hammes BJ, Cain JM. The ethics of pain management for cancer patients: case studies and analysis. J Pain Symptom Manage in press.

Hanks GW, Twycross RG, Lloyd JW. Unexpected complication of successful nerve block. Morphine induced respiratory depression precipitated by removal of severe pain. Anaesthesia 1981;36(1):37-9.

Hargreaves KM, Joris JL. The peripheral analgesic effects of opioids. APS Journal 1993;2(1):51-9.

Hayashi S. Der einfluss del ultraschallwellen und utrakurtzwellen auf den maligen tumor. Jpn J Med Sci Biophy 1940;6:138.

Health and Public Policy Committee, American College of Physicians. Drug therapy for severe, chronic pain in terminal illness. Ann Intern Med 1983;99(6):870-3.

Helig S. The San Francisco Medical Society Euthanasia Survey: results and analysis. SF Med 1988;61:24-34.

Hendler CS, Redd WH. Fear of hypnosis: the role of labeling in patients' acceptance of behavioral interventions. Behav Ther 1986;17(1):2-13.

Hendrickson M, Myre L, Johnson DG, Matlak ME, Black RE, Sullivan JJ. Postoperative analgesia in children: a prospective study in intermittent intramuscular injection versus continuous intravenous infusion of morphine. J Pediatr Surg 1990;25(2):185-91.

Hertzka RE, Gauntlett IS, Fisher DM, Spellman MJ. Fentanyl-induced ventilatory depression: effects of age. Anesthesiology 1989;70(2):213-8.

Hester NO. Comforting the child in pain. In: Funk SG, Tornquist EM, Champagne MT, Copp LA, Weise RA, editors. Key aspects of comfort:

management of pain, fatigue, and nausea. New York: Springer Publishing Co.; 1989. p. 290-8.

Hester NO, Barcus CS. Assessment and management of pain in children. Pediatr: Nurs Update 1986;1:1-8.

Hester NO, Foster R, Kristensen K. Measurement of pain in children: generalizability and validity of the Pain Ladder and the Poker Chip Tool. In: Tyler DC, Krane EJ, editors. Pediatric pain. Vol. 15. Advances in pain research and therapy. New York: Raven Press, Ltd.; 1990. p. 79-84.

Hester NO, Foster RL. Cues nurses and parents use in making judgments about children's pain. Pain 1990;(suppl. 5):S31.

Hester NO, Foster RL, Beyer JE. Clinical judgment in assessing children's pain. In: Watt-Watson JH, Donovan MI, editors. Pain management: nursing perspective. St. Louis: Mosby-Yearbook, Inc; 1992. p. 236-94.

Hester NO, Foster RL, Kristensen K, Bergstrom L. Measurement of children's pain by children, parents, and nurses: psychometric and clinical issues related to the Poker Chip Tool and the Pain Ladder. Final grant report. Generalizability of procedures assessing pain in children. 1989. Research funded by NIH, National Center for Nursing Research under Grant Number R23NRO1382, Sept. 1, 1986, through Aug. 31, 1988. [Available from N.O. Hester, Center for Nursing Research, School of Nursing, University of Colorado, Denver, CO 80262.]

Hill CS. A review and commentary on the negative influence of licensing and disciplinary boards and drug enforcement agencies on pain treatment with opioid analgesics. J Pharm Care in Pain & Symptom Control 1993;1(1):33-50.

Hill HF, Chapman CR, Kornell JA, Sullivan KM, Saeger LC, Bendetti C. Self-administration of morphine in bone marrow transplant patients reduces drug requirement. Pain 1990;40(2):121-9.

Hiraga K, Mizuguchi T, Takeda F. The incidence of cancer pain and improvement of pain management in Japan. Postgrad Med 1991;67(suppl.):S14-25.

Hodes RL. Cancer patients' needs and concerns when using narcotic analgesics. In: Hill CS Jr, Fields WS, editors. Drug treatment of cancer pain in a drug-oriented society. Vol. 11. Advances in pain research and therapy. New York: Raven Press, Ltd; 1989. p. 91-9.

Hodsman NB, Burns J, Blyth A, Kenny GN, McArdle CS, Rotman H. The morphine sparing effects of diclofenac sodium following abdominal surgery. Anaesthesia 1987;42(9):1005-8.

Hogan Q, Haddox JD, Abram S, Weissman D, Taylor ML, Janjan N. Epidural opiates and local anesthetics for the management of cancer pain. Pain 1991;46(3):271-9.

Holland JC, Rowland J, editors. Handbook of psychooncology: psychological care of the patient with cancer. New York: Oxford University Press; 1989.

Horan JJ, Laying FC, Pursell CH. Preliminary study of effects of "in vivo" emotive imagery on dental discomfort. Percept Mot Skills 1976;42(1):105-6.

Horowitz S, Patwardhan R, Marcus E. Hepatotoxic reactions associated with carbamazepine therapy. Epilepsia 1988;29(2):149-54.

Hoskin PJ. Scientific and clinical aspects of radiotherapy in the relief of bone pain. Cancer Surv 1988;7(1):69-86.

Houde RW. Methods for measuring clinical pain in humans. Acta Anaesthesiol Scand 1982;74(suppl.):25-9.

Houde RW. Analgesic effectiveness of the narcotic agonist-antagonists. Br J Clin Pharmac 1979;7:297S-308S.

Houde RW. The use and misuse of narcotics in the treatment of chronic pain. In: Bonica JJ, editor. International Symposium on Pain. Vol. 4 Advances in Neurology. New York: Raven Press, Ltd.; 1974. p. 527-36.

Howland JS, Baker MG, Poe T. Does patient education cause side effects? A controlled trial. J Fam Pract 1990;31(1):62-4.

International Association for the Study of Pain, Subcommittee on Taxonomy. Part II. Pain terms: a current list with definitions and notes on usage. Pain 1979;6:249-52 [updated 1982, 1986].

Inturrisi CE, Colburn WA, Kaiko RF, Houde RW, Foley KM. Pharmacokinetics and pharmacodynamics of methadone in patients with chronic pain. Clin Pharmacol Ther 1987;41:392-401.

Ischia S, Ischia A, Luzzani A, Toscano D, Steele A. Results up to death in the treatment of persistent cervico-thoracic (Pancoast) and thoracic malignant pain by unilateral percutaneous cervical cordotomy. Pain 1985;21 (4):339-55.

Ischia S, Ischia A, Polati E, Finco G. Three posterior percutaneous celiac plexus block techniques. A prospective, randomized study in 61 patients with pancreatic cancer pain. Anesthesiology 1992;76(4):534-40.

Ischia S, Luzzani A, Polati E. Retrogasserian glycerol injection: a retrospective study of 112 patients. Clin J Pain 1990;6(4):291-6.

Jacox A, Carr D, Payne R, et al. Managing Cancer Pain: Patient Guide. Clinical Practice Guideline Number 9 (Adult version—English). Rockville, MD: US Department of Health and Human Services, Public Health Service, Agency for Health Care Policy and Research. AHCPR Publication No. 93-0595, March 1994.

Jacox A, Carr D, Payne R, et al. Managing of Cancer Pain: Patient Guide. Clinical Practice Guideline Number 9 (Adult version—Spanish). Rockville, MD: US Department of Health and Human Services, Public Health Service, Agency for Health Care Policy and Research. AHCPR Publication No. 93-0596, in press.

Jaeckle KA, Young DF, Foley KM. The natural history of lumbosacral plexopathy in cancer. Neurology 1985;35(1):8-15.

Jaffe JH. Drug addiction and drug abuse. In: Gilman AG, Goodman LS, Rall TW, Murad F, editors. The pharmacological basis of therapeutics. 7th ed. New York: Macmillan Publishers; 1985. p. 532-81.

Janjan NA, Weissman DE, Pahule A. Improved pain management with daily nursing intervention during radiation therapy for head and neck carcinoma. Int J Radiat Oncol Biol Phys 1992;23(3):647-52.

Jay SM, Elliott CH, Ozolins M, Olson RA, Pruitt SD. Behavioral management of children's distress during painful medical procedures. Behav Res Ther 1985;23(5):513-20.

Jeff asks about cancer pain. Madison, WI: Wisconsin Cancer Pain Initiative; 1990. p. 12.

Johnson JE, Rice VH, Fuller SS, Endress MP. Sensory information, instruction in a coping strategy, and recovery from surgery. Res Nurs Health 1978;1(1):4-17.

Joranson DE. Federal and state regulation of opioids. J Pain Symptom Manage 1990;5(1 suppl.):S12-23.

Joranson DE. Are health care reimbursement policies a barrier to acute and cancer pain management? J Pain Symptom Manage in press.

Joranson DE, Cleeland CS, Weissman DE, Gilson AM. Opioids for chronic cancer and non-cancer pain: a survey of state medical board members. Federation Bulletin: The Journal of Medical Licensure and Discipline 1992;79(4):15-49.

Joshi JH, de Jongh CA, Schnaper N, Fortner CL, Wiernik PH. Amphetamine therapy for enhancing the comfort of terminally ill patients with cancer. 18th Annual Meeting of the American Society of Clinical Oncology; 1982 Apr 25-27; St. Louis. Proc Am Soc Clin Oncol 1982;1:55.

Kaiko RF. Age and morphine analgesia in cancer patients with post-operative pain. Clin Pharmacol Ther 1980;28(6):823-6.

Kaiko RF, Foley KM, Grabinski PY, Heidrich G, Rogers AG, Inturrisi CE, Reidenberg MM. Central nervous system excitatory effects of meperidine in cancer patients. Ann Neurol 1983;13(2):180-5.

Kaiko RF, Kanner R, Foley KM, Wallenstein SL, Canel AM, Rogers AG, Houde RW. Cocaine and morphine interaction in acute and chronic cancer pain. Pain 1987;31(1):35-45.

Kallos T, Caruso FS. Respiratory effects of butorphanol and pethidine. Anaesthesia 1979;34(7):633-7.

Kane RL, Ouslander JG, Abrass IB, editors. Essentials of clinical geriatrics. 2nd ed. New York: McGraw-Hill; 1989.

Kanner R. Post-surgical pain syndromes. In: Management of cancer pain: syllabus of the postgraduate course, Memorial Sloan-Kettering Cancer Center, 1985 Nov 14-16. New York: Memorial Sloan-Kettering Cancer Center; 1985. p. 65-72.

Kanner RM, Foley KM. Patterns of narcotic drug use in a cancer pain clinic. In: Research development in drug and alcohol use. Ann NY Acad Sci 1981;362:161-72.

Kanner RM, Portenoy RK. Unavailability of narcotic analgesics for ambulatory cancer patients in New York City. J Pain Symptom Manage 1986;1(2):87-9.

Kapelushnik J, Koren G, Solh H, Greenberg M, DeVeber L. Evaluating the efficacy of EMLA in alleviating pain associated with lumbar puncture; comparison of open and double-blinded protocols in children. Pain 1990;42(1):31-4.

Katz ER, Kellerman J, Ellenberg L. Hypnosis in the reduction of acute pain and distress in children with cancer. J Pediatr Psychol 1987;12(3):379-94.

Katz J, Levin AB. Treatment of diffuse metastatic cancer pain by instillation of alcohol into the sella turcica. Anesthesiology 1977;46(2):115-21.

Kaye BR. Rheumatologic manifestations of infection with human immunodeficiency virus (HIV). Ann Intern Med 1989;111(2):158-67.

Keller M. A retrospective review of patients receiving continuous morphine infusion. PRN Forum 1984;3:5-6.

Kelly JB, Payne R. Pain syndromes in the cancer patient. Neurol Clin 1991;9(4):937-53.

Kerr IG, Sone M, Deangelis C, Iscoe N, MacKenzie R, Schueller T. Continuous narcotic infusion with patient-controlled analgesia for chronic cancer pain in outpatients. Ann Intern Med 1988;108(4):554-7.

Khurana RC. Treatment of painful diabetic neuropathy with trazadone. JAMA 1983;250:1392.

Kishore-Kumar R, Max MB, Schafer SC, Gaughan AM, Smoller B, Gracely RH, Dubner R. Desipramine relieves postherpetic neuralgia. Clin Pharmacol Ther 1990;47(3):305-12.

Kisner C, Colby LA. Range of motion. In: Kisner C, Colby LA, editors. Therapeutic exercise: foundations and techniques. Philadelphia: FA Davis Co.; 1985. p. 19-65.

Koehntop DE, Rodman JH, Brundage DM, Hegland MG, Buckley JJ. Pharmacokinetics of fentanyl in neonates. Anesth Analg 1986;65(3):227-32.

Kohl HW, LaPorte RE, Blair SN. Physical activity and cancer. An epidemiological perspective. Sports Med 1988;6:222-37.

Kolassa M. Guidelines for clinicians in discerning and comparing the prices of pharmaceutical agents. J Pain Symptom Manage in press.

Koren G, Butt W, Chinyanga H, Soldin S, Tan YK, Pape K. Postoperative morphine infusion in newborn infants: assessment of disposition characteristics and safety. J Pediatr 1985;107(6):963-7.

Kori SH, Foley KM, Posner JB. Brachial plexus lesions in patients with cancer: 100 cases. Neurology 1981;31(1):45-50.

Kovar PA, Allegrante JP, MacKenzie R, Peterson MGE, Gutin B, Charlson ME. Supervised fitness walking in patients with osteoarthritis of the knee. A randomized, controlled trial. Ann Intern Med 1992;116(7):529-34.

Krames ES, Gershow J, Glassberg A, Kenefick T, Lyons A, Taylor P, Wilkie D. Continuous infusion of spinally administered narcotics for the relief of pain due to malignant disorders. Cancer 1985;56(3):696-702.

Kreek MJ, Garfield JW, Gutjahr CL, Giusti LM. Rifampin-induced methadone withdrawal. N Engl J Med 1976;294(20):1104-6.

Kuban DA, Schellhammer PF, el-Mahdi AM. Hemibody irradiation in advanced prostatic carcinoma. Urol Clin North Am 1991;18(1):131-7.

Kuttner L. Favorite stories: a hypnotic pain-reduction technique for children in acute pain. Am J Clin Hypn 1988;30(4):289-95.

Kvinesdal B, Molin J, Froland A, Gram LF. Imipramine treatment of painful diabetic neuropathy. JAMA 1984;251(13):1727-30.

Lahuerta J, Lipton S, Miles J, Wells CB. Update on percutaneous cervical cordotomy and pituitary alcohol neuroadenolysis: an audit of our recent results and complications. In: Lipton S, Miles J, editors. Persistent pain: modern methods of treatment. Vol 5. Orlando FL: Grune & Stratton; 1985. p. 197-223.

Lahuerta J, Lipton S, Wells JC. Percutaneous cervical cordotomy: results and complications in a recent series of 100 patients. Ann R Coll Surg Engl 1985;67(1):41-4.

Lasagna L, DeKornfeld TJ. Methotrimeprazine: a new phenothiazine derivative with analgesic properties. JAMA 1961;178(9):887-90.

Lawton PA, Maher EJ. Treatment strategies for advanced and metastatic cancer in Europe. Radiother Oncol 1991;22(1):1-6.

Lazorthes Y, Verdie JC, Bastide R, Lavados A, Descouens D. Spinal versus intraventricular chronic opiate administration with implantable drug delivery devices for cancer pain. Appl Neurophysiol 1985;48(1-6):234-41.

LeBaron S, Zeltzer L. Assessment of acute pain and anxiety in children and adolescents by self-reports, observer reports, and a behavior checklist. J Consult Clin Psychol 1984;52(5):729-38.

Lebovits AH, Lefkowitz M, McCarthy D, Simon R, Wilpon H, Jung R, Fried E. The prevalence and management of pain in patients with AIDS: a review of 134 cases. Clin J Pain 1989;5:245-8.

Lee MHM, Itoh M, Yang GW, Eason AL. Physical therapy and rehabilitation medicine. In: Bonica JJ, editor. The management of pain. 2nd ed. Vol. 2. Philadelphia: Lea & Febiger; 1990. p. 1769-88.

Lehmann JF, de Lateur BJ. Therapeutic heat. In: Lehmann JF, editor. Therapeutic heat and cold. 4th ed. Baltimore, MD: Williams & Wilkins; 1990. p. 417-581.

Lema MJ, Myers DP, de Leon-Casasola O, Penetrante R. Pleural phenol therapy for the treatment of chronic esophageal cancer pain. Reg Anesth 1992;17:166-70.

Lesko LM, Fleishman S. Treatment and support in confusional states. Recent Results Cancer Res 1991;121:378-92.

Levin AB, Katz J, Benson RC, Jones AG. Treatment of pain of diffuse metastatic cancer by stereotactic chemical hypophysectomy: long term results and observations on mechanism of action. Neurosurgery 1980;6(3):258-62.

Levin DN, Cleeland CS, Dar R. Public attitudes toward cancer pain. Cancer 1985;56(9):2337-9.

Levy MH. Integration of pain management into comprehensive cancer care. Cancer 1989;63:2328-35.

Levy MH. Constipation and diarrhea in cancer patients. Cancer Bull 1991;43(5):412-22.

Lewington VJ, McEwan AJ, Ackery DM, Bayly RJ, Keeling DH, Macleod PM, Porter AT, Zivanovic MA. A prospective, randomised double-blind crossover study to examine the efficacy of strontium-89 in pain palliation in patients with advanced prostate cancer metastatic to bone. Eur J Cancer 1991;27(8):954-8.

Lindstrom P, Lindblom U. The analgesic effect of tocainide in trigeminal neuralgia. Pain 1987;28:45-50.

Lipowski ZJ. Delirium (acute confusional states). JAMA 1987;258(13):1789-92.

Lipton S, Miles J, Williams N, Jones NB. Pituitary injection of alcohol for widespread cancer pain. Pain 1978;5(1):73-82.

Lynn AM, Slattery JT. Morphine pharmacokinetics in early infancy. Anesthesiology 1987;66(2):136-9.

Maher EJ, Coia L, Duncan G, Lawton PA. Treatment strategies in advanced and metastatic cancer: differences in attitude between the USA, Canada and Europe. Int J Radiat Oncol Biol Phys 1992;23(1):239-44.

Malawer MM, Delaney TF. Treatment of metastatic cancer to bone. In: DeVita VT Jr, Hellman S, Rosenberg SA, editors. Cancer: principles & practice of oncology. 3rd ed. Vol. 2. Philadelphia: JB Lippincott; 1989. p. 2298-316.

Maltbie AA, Cavenar JO Jr, Sullivan JL, Hammett EB, Zung WW. Analgesia and haloperidol: a hypothesis. J Clin Psychiatry 1979;40(7):323-6.

Mantell JE, Alexander ES, Kleiman MA. Social work and self-help groups. Health Soc Work 1976;1(1):86-100.

Marchand S. Nervous system stimulation for pain relief. APS Journal 1993;2(2):103-6.

Marks RM, Sachar EJ. Undertreatment of medical inpatients with narcotic analgesics. Ann Intern Med 1973;78(2):173-81.

Martin WR. Pharmacology of opioids. Pharmacol Rev 1984;35:283.

Massie MJ, Holland J, Glass E. Delirium in terminally ill cancer patients. Am J Psychiatry 1983;140(8):1048-50.

Massie MJ, Holland JC. Depression and the cancer patient. J Clin Psychiatry 1990;51(suppl.):12-17.

Massie MJ, Holland JC. The cancer patient with pain: psychiatric complications and their management. Med Clin North Am 1987;71(2):243-58.

Mastrovito R, Moynihan RT, Parsonnet L. Self-help and mutual support programs. In: Holland JC, Rowland JH, editors. Handbook of psychooncology: psychological care of the patient with cancer. New York: Oxford University Press; 1989. p. 502-7.

Maves TJ, Gebhart GF. Antinociceptive synergy between intrathecal morphine and lidocaine during visceral and somatic nociception in the rat. Anesthesiology 1992;76:91-9.

Max MB. Improving outcomes of analgesic treatment: is education enough? Ann Intern Med 1990;113(11):885-9.

Max MB, Culnane M, Schafer SC, Gracely RH, Walther DJ, Smoller B, Dubner R. Amitriptyline relieves diabetic neuropathy pain in patients with normal or depressed mood. Neurology 1987;37(4):589-96.

Max MB, Inturrisi CE, Kaiko RF, Grabinski PY, Li CH, Foley KM. Epidural and intrathecal opiates: cerebrospinal fluid and plasma profiles in patients with chronic cancer pain. Clin Pharmacol Ther 1985;38:631-41.

Max MB, Schafer SC, Culnane M, Smoller B, Dubner R, Gracely RH. Amitriptyline, but not lorazepam, relieves postherpetic neuralgia. Neurology 1988;38(9):1427-32.

Maxon HR III, Schroder LE, Thomas SR, Hertzberg VS, Deutsch EA, Scher HI, Samaratunga RC, Libson KF, Williams CC, Moulton JS, Schneider HJ. Re-186(Sn) HEDP for treatment of osseous metastases: initial clinical experience in 20 patients with hormone-resistant prostate cancer. Radiology 1990;176(1):155-9.

Maxon HR III, Smith HS. Radioiodine-131 in the diagnosis and treatment of metastatic well-differentiated thyroid cancer. Endocrinol Metab Clin North Am 1990;19(3):685-718.

Mayer DJ, Liebeskind JC. Pain reduction by focal electrical stimulation of the brain: an anatomical and behavioral analysis. Brain Res 1974;68:73-93.

Mayer DK. Non-pharmacologic management of pain in the person with cancer. J Adv Nurs 1985;10(4):325-30.

McCaffery M, Beebe A. Pain: clinical manual for nursing practice. St. Louis: CV Mosby Co.; 1989.

McCaffery M, Martin L, Ferrell BR. Analgesic administration via rectum or stoma. ET Nurs 1992;19(4):114-21.

McCaffery M, Wolff M. Pain relief using cutaneous modalities, positioning, and movement. In: Turk DC, Feldman CS, editors. Special issue: noninvasive approaches to pain management in the terminally ill. Hospice J 1992;8(1-2):121-53. New York: Haworth Press.

McCaul KD, Malott JM. Distraction and coping with pain. Psychol Bull 1984;95(3):516-33.

McGivney WT, Crooks GM. The care of patients with severe chronic pain in terminal illness. JAMA 1984;251(9):1182-8.

McGrath PA. The plasticity and complexity of the nociceptive system. In: McGrath PA, editor. Pain in children: nature, assessment, and treatment. New York: The Guilford Press; 1990a. p. 88-110.

McGrath PA, editor. Pain in children: nature, assessment, and treatment. New York: The Guilford Press; 1990b.

McGrath PA, de Veber LL, Hearn MT. Multidimensional pain assessment in children. In: Fields HL, Dubner R, Cervero F, editors. Proceedings of the Fourth World Congress on Pain, Seattle. Vol. 9. Advances in pain research and therapy. New York: Raven Press, Ltd.; 1985. p. 387-93.

McGrath PJ, Unruh AM. Pain in children and adolescents. New York: Elsevier Science Publishers; 1987.

McKinney's Public Health Law, sec. 3302 (1).

Meglio M, Cioni B. Personal experience with spinal cord stimulation in chronic pain management. In: Gildenberg PL, et al., editors. Proceedings of the eighth meeting of the World society and fifth meeting of the European society, Zurich, Switzerland, July 9-11, 1981. Stereotactic and functional neurosurgery. Vol. 9. Advances in stereoencephalotomy. New York: S. Karger; 1982. p. 195-200.

Meglio M, Cioni B, Rossi GF. Spinal cord stimulation in management of chronic pain. A 9-year experience. J Neurosurg 1989;70(4):519-24.

Meignier M, Souron R, Le Neel JC. Postoperative dorsal epidural analgesia in the child with respiratory disabilities. Anesthesiology 1983;59(5):473-5.

Melding PS. Is there such a thing as geriatric pain? Pain 1991;46(2):119-21.

Melzack R. The tragedy of needless pain. Sci Am 1990;262(2):27-33.

Mercadante S. Celiac plexus block versus analgesics in pancreatic cancer pain. Pain 1993;52:187-92.

Messerli ML, Garamendi C, Romano J. Breast cancer: information as a technique of crisis intervention. Am J Orthopsychiatry 1980;50(4):728-31.

Meyerson BA. Central nervous stimulation for cancer pain: possible methods of manipulating the physiology of pain control. In: Bonica JJ, Ventafridda V, Pagni CA, editors. Management of superior pulmonary sulcus syndrome (Pancoast Syndrome). Vol. 4, Advances in pain research and therapy. New York: Raven Press, Ltd.; 1982. p. 149-64.

Meyerson BA, Boethius J, Carlsson AM. Percutaneous central gray stimulation for cancer pain. Appl Neurophysiol 1978;41(1-4):57-65.

Miaskowski C, Donovan M. Implementation of the American Pain Society Quality Assurance Standards for Relief of Acute Pain and Cancer Pain in oncology nursing practice. Oncol Nurs Forum 1992;19(3):411-5.

Miaskowski C, Jacox A, Hester NO, Ferrell B. Interdisciplinary guidelines for the management of acute pain: implications for quality improvement. J Nurs Care Qual 1992;7(1):1-6.

Michlovitz SL. Diathermy and pulsed electromagnetic fields. In: Michlovitz SL, editor. Thermal agents in rehabilitation. 2nd ed. Philadelphia: FA Davis and Co.; 1990.

Middaugh SJ, Levin RB, Kee WG, Barchiesi FD, Roberts JM. Chronic pain: its treatment in geriatric and younger patients. Arch Phys Med Rehabil 1988;69(12):1021-6.

Miles J, Lipton S, Hayward M, Bowsher D, Mumford J, Molony V. Pain relief by implanted electrical stimulators. Lancet 1974;1(861):777-9.

Miser AW. Management of pain associated with childhood cancer. In: Schechter NL, Berde CB, Yaster M, editors. Pain in infants, children, and adolescents. Baltimore: Williams & Wilkins; 1993. p. 411-24.

Miser AW, Ayesh D, Broda E, McCalla J, Steinberg SM, Wall R, Jelenich S, Lees DE, Wilkinson TK, Miser JS. Use of a patient-controlled device for nitrous oxide administration to control procedure-related pain in children and young adults with cancer. Pain 1988;4:5-10.

Miser AW, Dothage JA, Wesley RA, Miser JS. The prevalence of pain in a pediatric and young adult cancer population. Clin J Pain 1987;29(1):73-83.

Miser AW, Miser JS. The use of oral methadone to control moderate and severe pain in children and young adults with malignancy. Clin J Pain 1986;1:243-8.

Miser AW, Miser JS. The treatment of cancer pain in children. Pediatr Clin North Am 1989;36(4):979-99.

Miser AW, Moore L, Greene R, Gracely RH, Miser JS. Prospective study of continuous intravenous and subcutaneous morphine infusions for therapy-related or cancer-related pain in children and young adults with cancer. Clin J Pain 1986;2:101-6.

Mishel MH. Perceived uncertainty and stress in illness. Res Nurs Health 1984;7(3):163-71.

Moinpour CM, Chapman CR. Pain management and quality of life in cancer patients. In: Lehmann RKA, Zech D, editors. Transdermal fentanyl: a new approach to prolonged pain control. Berlin: Springer-Verlag; 1991. p. 42-63.

Morris HG, Sherman NA, McQuain C, Goldlust MB, Chang SF, Harrison LI. Effects of salsalate (nonacetylated salicylate) and aspirin on serum prostaglandins in humans. Ther Drug Monit 1985;7:435-8.

Moulin DE, Kreeft JH, Murray-Parsons N, Bouquillon AI. Comparison of continuous subcutaneous and intravenous hydromorphone infusion for management of cancer pain. Lancet 1991;337(8739):465-8.

Munro S, Mount B. Music therapy in palliative care. Can Med Assoc J 1978;119(9);1029-34.

Nagashima H, Karamanian A, Malovany R, Radnay P, Ang M, Koerner S, Foldes FF. Respiratory and circulatory effects of intravenous butorphanol and morphine. Clin Pharmacol Ther 1976;19(6):738-45.

Nahata MC, Clotz MA, Krogg EA. Adverse effects of meperidine, promethazine, and chlorpromazine for sedation in pediatric patients. Clin Pediatr (Phila) 1985;24(10):558-60.

Nahata MC, Miser AW, Miser JS, Reuning RH. Analgesic plasma concentrations of morphine in children with terminal malignancy receiving a continuous subcutaneous infusion of morphine sulfate to control severe pain. Pain 1984;18(2):109-14.

National Cancer Institute. NCI Workshop on Cancer Pain. Sept 14-15, 1990; Bethesda, MD.

National Institutes of Health Consensus Development Conference. The integrated approach to the management of pain. J Pain Symptom Manage 1987;2(1):35-44.

Newman RG. The need to redefine "addiction." N Engl J Med 1983;308 (18):1096-8.

Nielsen OS, Munro AJ, Tannock IF. Bone metastases: pathophysiology and management policy. J Clin Oncol 1991;9(3):509-24.

Nittner K. Stimulation of conus-epiconus with pisces—further indications. Acta Neurochir (Wien) 1980;(suppl.) 30:311-6.

North RB. The role of spinal cord stimulation in contemporary pain management. APS Journal 1993;2(2):91-9.

The Nurses' Association of the American College of Obstetricians and Gynecologists (NAACOG) Committee on Practice. OGN nursing practice resource. Prevention, recognition, and management of neonatal pain. Washington, DC: NAACOG; April 1991. Available from: NAACOG; The Organization for Obstetric, Gynecologic, and Neonatal Nurses; 409 12th St., S.W.; Washington, DC 20024-2191.

O'Neill WM, Sherrard JS. Pain in human immune deficiency virus disease: a review. Pain 1993;54:3-14.

O'Young J, McPeek B. Quality of life variables in surgical trials. J Chron Dis 1987;40(6):513-22.

Obbens EA, Hill CS, Leavens ME, Ruthenbeck SS, Otis F. Intraventricular morphine administration for control of chronic cancer pain. Pain 1987;28(1):61-8.

Oda MAS, Schurman DJ. Monitoring of pathological fracture. In: Stoll BA, Parbhoo S, editors. Bone metastasis: monitoring and treatment. New York: Raven Press, Ltd.; 1983. p. 271-88.

Olness K. Hypnosis in pediatric practice. Curr Probl Pediatr 1981;12(2):1-47.

Onghena P, Van Houdenhove B. Antidepressant-induced analgesia in chronic non-malignant pain: a meta-analysis of 39 placebo-controlled studies. Pain 1992;49(2):205-19.

Onofrio BM, Yaksh TL. Long-term pain relief produced by intrathecal morphine infusion in 53 patients. J Neurosurg 1990;72:200-9.

Paice J. Personal communication. May 5, 1993.

Paice J. Resources in cancer pain management. Oncol Nurs Forum 1990;17(4):587-90.

Patchell RA, Posner JB. Cancer and the nervous system. In: Holland JC, Rowland JH, editors. The handbook of psychooncology: psychological care of the patient with cancer. New York: Oxford University Press; 1989. p. 327-41.

Patel M, Gutzwiller F, Paccaud F, Marazzi A. A meta-analysis of acupuncture for chronic pain. Int J Epidemiol 1989;18(4):900-6.

Patt RB. Cancer pain. Philadelphia: JB Lippincott Co.; 1993.

Payne R. Transdermal fentanyl: suggested recommendations for clinical use. J Pain Symptom Manage 1992;7(suppl. 3):S40-4.

Payne RC. Post-chemotherapy and post-radiation therapy pain syndromes. In: Management of cancer pain: syllabus of the postgraduate course, Memorial Sloan-Kettering Cancer Center, 1985 Nov 14-16. New York: Memorial Sloan-Kettering Cancer Center; 1985. p. 73-93.

Pellock JM. Carbamazepine side effects in children and adults. Epilepsia 1987;28(suppl. 3):S64-S70.

Pfaff VK, Smith KE, Gowan D. The effects of music-assisted relaxation on the distress of pediatric cancer patients undergoing bone marrow aspirations. Child Health Care 1989;18(4):232-6.

Pfalzer L. Physical agents and the patient with cancer. Clin Manage Phys Ther 1992;12(4):83-6.

Pilowsky I, Hallett EC, Bassett DL, Thomas PG, Penhall RK. A controlled study of amitriptyline in the treatment of chronic pain. Pain 1982;14(2):169-79.

Popkin MK, Callies AL, Mackenzie TB. The outcome of antidepressant use in the medically ill. Arch Gen Psychiatry 1985;42(12):1160-3.

Portenoy RK. Continuous infusion of opioid drugs in the treatment of cancer pain: guidelines for use. J Pain Symptom Manage 1986;1(4):223-8.

Portenoy RK. Continuous intravenous infusion of opioid drugs. Med Clin North Am 1987;71(2):233-41.

Portenoy RK. Personal communication. June 15, 1993.

Portenoy RK. Practical aspects of pain control in the patient with cancer. CA Cancer J Clin 1988;38(6):327-52.

Portenoy RK, Hagen NA. Breakthrough pain: definition, prevalence and characteristics. Pain 1990;41(3):273-81.

Portenoy RK, Lipton RB, Foley KM. Back pain in the cancer patient: an algorithm for evaluation and management. Neurology 1987;37(1):134-8.

Portenoy RK, Payne R. Acute and chronic pain. In: Lowinson JH, Ruiz P, Millman RB, editors. Substance abuse: a comprehensive textbook. 2nd ed. Baltimore: Williams & Wilkins; 1992. p. 691-721.

Portenoy RK, Southam MA, Gupta SK, Lapin J, Layman M, Inturrisi CE, Foley KM. Transdermal fentanyl for cancer pain. Repeated dose pharmacokinetics. Anesthesiology 1993;78(1):36-43.

Poulter CA, Cosmatos D, Rubin P, Urtasun R, Cooper JS, Kuske RR, Hornback N, Coughlin C, Weigensberg I, Rotman M. A report of RTOG 8206: a phase III study of whether the addition of single dose hemibody irradiation to standard fractionated local field irradiation is more effective than local field irradiation alone in the treatment of symptomatic osseous metastases. Int J Radiat Oncol Biol Phys 1992;23(1):207-14.

Powell KE, Thompson PD, Caspersen CJ, Kendrick JS. Physical activity and the incidence of coronary heart disease. Annu Rev Public Health 1987;8:253-87.

Price P, Hoskin PJ, Easton D, Austin D, Palmer SG, Yarnold JR. Prospective randomised trial of single and multifraction radiotherapy schedules in the treatment of painful bony metastases. Radiother Oncol 1986;6(4):247-55.

Puntillo KA. Pain experiences of intensive care unit patients. Heart Lung 1990;19(5 Pt 1):526-33.

Purcell-Jones G, Dormon F, Sumner E. The use of opioids in neonates. A retrospective study of 933 cases. Anaesthesia 1987;42(12):1316-20.

Raj PP. Practical management of pain. 2nd ed. St. Louis: Mosby Year Book; 1992.

Rawal M, Möllefors K, Axelsson K, Lingårdh G, Widman B. An experimental study of urodynamic effects of epidural morphine and of naloxone reversal. Anesth Analg 1983;62:641-7.

Reading AE. The effects of psychological preparation on pain and recovery after minor gynecological surgery: preliminary report. J Clin Psychol 1982;38(3):504-12.

Reeves JL, Redd WH, Storm FK, Minagawa RY. Hypnosis in the control of pain during hyperthermia treatment of cancer. In: Bonica JJ, Lindblom U, Iggo A, editors. Proceedings of the Third World Congress on Pain, Edinburgh. Vol. 5. Advances in pain research and therapy. New York: Raven Press, Ltd.; 1983. p. 857-61.

Reich W. Encyclopedia of bioethics. New York: The Free Press; 1992.

Reynolds DV. Surgery in the rat during electrical analgesia induced by focal brain stimulation. Science 1969;164:444-5.

Rhiner M, Ferrell BR, Ferrell BA, Grant MM. A structured non-drug intervention program for cancer pain. Cancer Practice 1993;1(2):137-43.

Rimer B, Levy MH, Keintz MK, Fox L, Engstrom PF, MacElwee N. Enhancing cancer pain control regimens through patient education. Patient Educ Couns 1987;10(3):267-77.

Robinson RG, Spicer JA, Preston DR, Wegst AV, Martin NL. Treatment of metastatic bone pain with strontium-89. Int J Rad Appl Instrum [B] 1987;14(3):219-22.

Rodriguez M, Dinapoli RP. Spinal cord compression: with special reference to metastatic epidural tumors. Mayo Clin Proc 1980;55(7):442-8.

Rodriguez-Bigas M, Petrelli NJ, Herrera L, West C. Intrathecal phenol rhizotomy for management of pain in recurrent unresectable carcinoma of the rectum. Surg Gynecol Obstet 1991;173(1):41-4.

Rogers AG. The use of methotrimeprazine (Levoprome) in a patient sensitive to opioids and possible bowel shutdown. J Pain Symptom Manage 1989;4(1):44-5.

Ross DM. Thought-stopping: a coping strategy for impending feared events. Issues Compr Pediatr Nurs 1984;7(2-3):83-9.

Ross DM, Ross SA. Childhood pain: current issues, research, and management. Baltimore: Urban & Schwarzenberg; 1988.

Roth A, Kolaric K. Analgetic activity of calcitonin in patients with painful osteolytic metastases of breast cancer. Oncology 1986;43:283-7.

Roth SH. Merits and liabilities of NSAID therapy. Rheum Dis Clin North Am 1989;15(3):479-98.

Rusthoven JJ, Ahlgren P, Elhakim T, Pinfold P, Reid J, Stewart L, Feld R. Varicella-zoster infection in adult cancer patients. A population study. Arch Intern Med 1988;148(7):1561-6.

Ryan EA. The effect of musical distraction on pain in hospitalized school-aged children. In: Funk SG, Tornquist EM, Champagne MT, Copp LA, Wiese RA, editors. Key aspects of comfort: management of pain, fatigue, and nausea. New York: Springer Publishing Co.; 1989. p. 101-4.

Salazar OM, Rubin P, Hendrickson FR, Komaki R, Poulter C, Newall J, Asbell SO, Mohiuddin M, van Ess J. Single dose half-body irradiation for palliation of multiple bone metastases from solid tumors. Final Radiation Therapy Oncology Group report. Cancer 1986;58(1):29-36.

Salmon JB, Finch PM, Lovegrove FT, Warwick A. Mapping of spread of epidural phenol in cancer pain patients by radionuclide admixture and epidural scintigraphy. Clin J Pain 1992;8:18-22.

Savedra MC, Tesler MD, Holzemer WL, Ward JA. Adolescent Pediatric Pain Tool (APPT) preliminary user's manual. San Francisco: University of California; 1989; updated 1992. [Available from M.C. Savedra, UCSF School of Nursing, San Francisco, CA 94143-0606.]

Savedra MC, Tesler MD, Holzemer WL, Wilkie DJ, Ward JA. Pain location: validity and reliability of body outline markings by hospitalized children and adolescents. Res Nurs Health 1989;12(5):307-14.

Schechter NL. The undertreatment of pain in children: an overview. Pediatr Clin North Am 1989;36(4):781-94.

Schechter NL, Weisman SJ, Rosenblum M, Beck A, Altman A, Quinn J, Conrad PF. Sedation for painful procedures in children with cancer using the fentanyl lollipop: a preliminary report. In: Tyler DC, Krane EJ, editors. Pediatric pain. Vol. 15. Advances in pain research and therapy. New York: Raven Press, Ltd.; 1990. p. 209-214.

Schlegel SI. General characteristics of nonsteroidal anti-inflammatory drugs. In: Paulus HE, Furst DE, Dromgoole SH, editors. Anti-inflammatory agents, non-steroidal. Vol. 16. Drugs for rheumatic disease. New York: Churchill Livingstone; 1987. p. 203-26.

Schofferman J, Brody R. Pain in far advanced AIDS. In: Foley KM, Bonica JJ, Ventafridda V, editors. Proceedings of the Second International Congress on Cancer Pain. Vol. 16. Advances in pain research and therapy. New York: Raven Press, Ltd.; 1990. p. 379-86.

Schug SA, Zech D, Dörr U. Cancer pain management according to WHO analgesic guidelines. J Pain Symptom Manage 1990;5(1):27-32.

Schvarcz JR. Spinal cord stereotactic techniques re: trigeminal nucleotomy and extralemniscal myelotomy. Appl Neurophysiol 1978;41(1-4):99-112.

Sear JW, Hand CW, Moore RA, McQuay HJ. Studies on morphine disposition: influence of renal failure on the kinetics of morphine and its metabolites. Br J Anaesth 1989;62(1):28-32.

Shapiro RS. Legal bases for control of analgesic drugs. J Pain Symptom Manage in press.

Shapiro RS. Liability issues in the management of pain. J Pain Symptom Manage in press.

Sherry MM, Greco FA, Johnson DH, Hainsworth JD. Breast cancer with skeletal metastases at initial diagnosis. Distinctive clinical characteristics and favorable prognosis. Cancer 1986a;58(1):178-82.

Sherry MM, Greco FA, Johnson DH, Hainsworth JD. Metastatic breast cancer confined to the skeletal system. An indolent disease. Am J Med 1986b;81(3):381-6.

Siegel LJ, Peterson L. Maintenance effects of coping skills and sensory information on young children's response to repeated dental procedures. Behav Ther 1981;12(4):530-5.

Sievers TD, Yee JD, Foley ME, Blanding PJ, Berde CB. Midazolam for conscious sedation during pediatric oncology procedures: safety and recovery parameters. Pediatrics 1991;88(6):1172-9.

Silberstein EB. Review of efficacy of strontium 89 therapy. Unpublished manuscript.

Silberstein EB, Elgazzar AH, Kapilivsky A. Phosphorus-32 radiopharmaceuticals for the treatment of painful osseous metastases. Semin Nucl Med 1992;22(1):17-27.

Silberstein EB, Williams C. Strontium-89 therapy for the pain of osseous metastases. J Nucl Med 1985;26(4):345-8.

Sindou M, Fischer G, Goutelle A, Allegre GE. Micro surgical selective posterior rhizotomy. 69 cases. Third World Congress on Pain, Edinburgh, Scotland, Sept 4-11, 1981. Pain 1981;(suppl. 1):S289.

Singer EJ, Zorilla C, Fahy-Chandon B, Chi S, Syndulko K, Tourtellotte WW. Painful symptoms reported by ambulatory HIV-infected men in a longitudinal study. Pain 1993;54(1):15-9.

Siscovick DS, LaPorte RE, Newman JM. The disease-specific benefits and risks of physical activity and exercise. Public Health Rep 1985;100:180-8.

Sjölund BH, Eriksson MBE. Endorphins and analgesia produced by peripheral conditioning stimulation. In: Bonica JJ, Liebeskind DG, Albe-Fessard D, editors. Proceedings of the Second World Congress on Pain, Montreal, Quebec. Vol. 3. Advances in pain research and therapy. New York: Raven Press, Ltd.; 1979. p. 587-92.

Smith JA. Palliation of painful bone metastases from prostate cancer using sodium etidronate: results of a randomized, prospective, double-blind, placebo-controlled study. J Urol 1989;141:85-87.

Sorkin BA, Rudy TE, Hanlon RB, Turk DC, Stieg RL. Chronic pain in old and young patients: differences appear less important than similarities. J Gerontol 1990;45(2):P64-8.

Spiegel D, Bloom JR. Group therapy and hypnosis reduce metastatic breast carcinoma pain. Psychosom Med 1983;45(4):333-9.

Spiegel D, Bloom JR, Kraemer HC, Gottheil E. Effect of psychosocial treatment on survival of patients with metastatic breast cancer. Lancet 1989;2(8668):888-91.

Spiegel K, Kalb R, Pasternak GW. Analgesic activity of tricyclic antidepressants. Ann Neurol 1983;13(4):462-5.

Spross JA. The CNS as collaborator. In: Hamric AB, Spross JA, editors. The clinical nurse specialist in theory and practice. 2nd ed. Philadelphia: WB Saunders Co.; 1989. p. 205-26.

Spross JA, McGuire DB, Schmitt RM. Oncology Nursing Society Position Paper on Cancer Pain. Part I: introduction and background. Oncol Nurs Forum 1990a;17(4):595-614.

Spross JA, McGuire DB, Schmitt RM. Oncology Nursing Society Position Paper on Cancer Pain. Part II: education. Oncol Nurs Forum 1990b; 17(5):751-60.

Spross JA, McGuire DB, Schmitt RM. Oncology Nursing Society Position Paper on Cancer Pain. Part III: nursing administration. Oncol Nurs Forum 1990c;17(6):944-5.

Sriwatanakul K, Kelvie W, Lasagna L. The quantification of pain: an analysis of words used to describe pain and analgesia in clinical trials. Clin Pharmacol Ther 1982;32(2):143-8.

Stein C. Peripheral mechanisms of opioid analgesia. Anesth Analg 1993;76 (1):182-91.

Stiefel F, Holland J. Delirium in cancer patients. International Psychogeriatrics 1991;3(2):222-6.

Stiefel FC, Breitbart WS, Holland JC. Corticosteroids in cancer: neuropsychiatric complications. Cancer Invest 1989;7(5):479-91.

Stjernsward J, Teoh N. The scope of the cancer pain problem. In: Foley KM, Bonica JJ, Ventafridda V, editors. Proceedings of the Second International Congress on Cancer Pain; 1988; Rye, NY. Vol. 16. Advances in pain research and therapy. New York: Raven Press, Ltd.; 1990. p. 7-12.

Stover J. Cancer pain: A patient's view. Unpublished manuscript February 1992.

Stuart JJ, Pisko EJ. Choline magnesium trisalicylate does not impair platelet aggregation. Pharmatherapeutica 1981;2(8):547-51.

Stuart MJ, Murphy S, Oski FA, Evans AE, Donaldson MH, Gardner FH. Platelet function in recipients of platelets from donors ingesting aspirin. N Engl J Med 1972;287(22):1105-9.

Sunshine A, Olson NZ. Non-narcotic analgesics. In: Wall PD, Melzack R, editors. Textbook of Pain. 2nd Ed. New York: Churchill Livingstone; 1989. p. 670-85.

Sutor AH, Bowie EJ, Owen CA Jr. Effect of aspirin, sodium salicylate, and acetaminophen on bleeding. Mayo Clin Proc 1971;46(3):178-81.

Swanson G, Smith J, Bulich R, New P, Shiffman R. Patient-controlled analgesia for chronic cancer pain in the ambulatory setting: a report of 117 patients. J Clin Oncol 1989;7(12):1903-8.

Sweet WH. Treatment of facial pain by percutaneous differential thermal trigeminal rhizotomy. Prog Neurol Surg 1976;7:153-79.

Swerdlow M. Anticonvulsant drugs and chronic pain. Clin Neuropharmacol 1984;7(1):51-82.

Swerdlow M. Role of chemical neurolysis and local anesthetic infiltration. In: Swerdlow M, Ventafridda V, editors. Cancer pain. Lancaster: MTP Press; 1987.

Syrjala KL. Integrating medical and psychological treatments for cancer pain. In: Chapman CR, Foley KM, editors. Current and emerging issues in cancer pain: research and practice. New York: Raven Press, Ltd.; in press.

Syrjala KL. Relaxation techniques. In: Bonica JJ, editor. The management of pain. 2nd ed. Vol. II. Philadelphia: Lea & Febiger; 1990. p. 1742-50.

Syrjala KL, Cummings C, Donaldson GW. Hypnosis or cognitive behavioral training for the reduction of pain and nausea during cancer treatment: a controlled clinical trial. Pain 1992;48(2):137-46.

Szeto HH, Inturrisi CE, Houde R, Saal S, Cheigh J, Reidenberg MM. Accumulation of normeperidine, an active metabolite of meperidine, in patients with renal failure of cancer. Ann Intern Med 1977;86(6):738-41.

Takeda F. Results of field-testing in Japan of the WHO draft interim guidelines on relief of cancer pain. Pain Clin 1986;1:83-9.

Takeda F, Fujii T, Uki J, Fuse Y, Tozawa R, Kitani Y, Fujita T. Cancer pain relief and tumor regression by means of pituitary neuroadenolysis and surgical hypophysectomy. Neurol Med Chir (Tokyo) 1983;23(1):41-9.

Tasker RR. Percutaneous cordotomy: the lateral high cervical technique. In: Schmidek HH, Sweet WH, editors. Operative neurosurgical techniques: indications, methods, and results. 2nd ed. Vol. 2. Philadelphia: WB Saunders Co.; 1988. p. 1191-205.

Teamwork: the cancer patient's guide to talking with your doctor. Silver Spring, MD: National Coalition for Cancer Survivorship; 1991. p. 32.

Tejwani GA, Rattan AK, McDonald JS. Role of spinal opioid receptors in the antinociceptive interactions between intrathecal morphine and bupivacaine. Anesth Analg 1992;74:726-34.

Tennant FS Jr, Uelmen GF. Prescribing narcotics to habitual and addicted narcotics users. Medical and legal guidelines in California and some other Western states. West J Med 1980;133(6):539-45.

Teoh N, Stjernsward J. WHO cancer pain relief program—ten years on. Seattle: International Association for the Study of Pain, IASP Newsletter 1992; p. 5-6.

ter Riet G, Kleijnen J, Knipschild P. Acupuncture and chronic pain: a criteria-based meta-analysis. J Clin Epidemiol 1990;43(11):1191-9.

Tesler MD, Savedra MC, Holzemer WL, Wilkie DJ, Ward JA, Paul SM. The word-graphic rating scale as a measure of children's and adolescents' pain intensity. Res Nurs Health 1991;14(5):361-71.

Thames HD, Withers HR, Peters LJ, Fletcher GH. Changes in early and late radiation responses with altered dose fractionation: implications for dose-survival relationships. Int J Rad Biol Phys 1982;8:219-26.

Thangathurai D, Bowles HF, Allen HW, Mikhail M. The incidence of pruritus after epidural morphine (letter). Anaesthesia 1988;43(12):1055-6.

Tobias JD. Pediatric pain management: the use of non-narcotic analgesic agents. Analgesia: J Pain Ther Health Care Prof 1992;3(3):4-6.

Todd KH, Samaroo N, Hoffman JR. Ethnicity as a risk factor for inadequate emergency department analgesia. JAMA 1993;269(12):1537-9.

Tong D, Gillick L, Hendrickson FR. The palliation of symptomatic osseous metastases: final results of the Study by the Radiation Therapy Oncology Group. Cancer 1982;50(5):893-9.

Turkington RM. Depression masquerading as diabetic neuropathy. JAMA 1980;243:1147-50.

Turner JH, Claringbold PG, Hetherington EL, Sorby P, Martindale AA. A phase I study of samarium-153 ethylenediaminetetramethylene phosphonate therapy for disseminated skeletal metastases. J Clin Oncol 1989;7(12):1926-31.

Twycross RG. Choice of strong analgesic in terminal cancer: diamorphine or morphine? Pain 1977;3:93-104.

Uniform Controlled Substances Act (1990), U.L.A. Vol. 9, Part II sec 101 et seq.

US Department of Health and Human Services, Agency for Health Care Policy and Research. Public Meeting on Clinical Practice Guidelines for

Cancer-Related Pain. Federal Register July 31, 1991. Vol. 56(147):36155-36156, and Federal Register Aug 20, 1991. Vol. 56(161):41391.

van Dongen RT, Crul BJ. Paraplegia following coeliac plexus block. Anaesthesia 1991;46(10):862-3.

van Holten-Verzantvoort ATM, Zwinderman AH, Aaronson NK, Hermans J, van Emmerik B, van Dam FS, van den Bos B, Bijvoet OL, Cleton FJ. The effect of supportive pamidronate treatment on aspects of quality of life of patients with advanced breast cancer. Eur J Cancer 1991;27:544-549.

van Roost D, Gybels J. Myelotomies for chronic pain. Acta Neurochir Suppl (Wien) 1989;46:69-72.

Varvel JR, Shafer SL, Hwang SS, Coen PA, Stanski DR. Absorption characteristics of transdermally administered fentanyl. Anesthesiology 1989;70(6):928-34.

Vasudevan S, Hegmann K, Moore A, Cerletty S. Physical methods of pain management. In: Raj PP, editor. Practical management of pain. 2nd ed. Baltimore: Mosby Year Book Medical Publishers; 1992. p. 669-79.

Ventafridda V, Bianchi M, Ripamonti C, Sacerdote P, De Conno F, Zecca E, Panerai AE. Studies on the effects of antidepressant drugs on the antinociceptive action of morphine and on plasma morphine in rat and man. Pain 1990;43(2):155-62.

Ventafridda V, Bonezzi C, Caraceni A, De Conno F, Guarise G, Ramella G, Saita L, Silvani V, Tamburini M, Toscani F. Antidepressants for cancer pain and other painful syndromes with deafferentation component: comparison of amitriptyline and trazodone. Ital. J Neurol Sci 1987;8(6):579-87.

Ventafridda V, Caraceni A, Gamba A. Field-testing of the WHO Guidelines for Cancer Pain Relief: summary report of demonstration projects. In: Foley KM, Bonica JJ, Ventafridda V, editors. Proceedings of the Second International Congress on Pain. Vol. 16. Advances in pain research and therapy. New York: Raven Press, Ltd.; 1990. p. 451-64.

Ventafridda GV, Caraceni AT, Sbanotto AM, Barletta L, De Conno F. Pain treatment in cancer of the pancreas. Eur J Surg Oncol 1990;16:1-6.

Verrill PJ. Adverse effects and complications of stellate lumbar and splanchnic sympathetic blocks with neurolytic preparations. In: Mumenthaler M, Van Zwieten PA, Farcot JM, editors. Treatment of chronic pain: possibilities, limitations and long-term follow-up. New York: Harwood Academic Publishers; 1990. p. 127-33.

Von Roenn JH, Cleeland CS, Gonin R, Hatfield AK, Pandya KJ. Physician attitudes and practice in cancer pain management: a survey from the Eastern Cooperative Oncology Group. Ann Intern Med 1993;119(2):121-6.

Wagner G. Frequency of pain in patients with cancer. Recent Results Cancer Res 1984;89:64-71.

Waldman SD. Acute herpes zoster involving the chest wall. In: Ferrer-Brechner T. Common problems in pain management. Littleton, Mass: Year Book Medical Publishers, Inc.; 1990. p. 143-51.

Walker KN, MacBride A, Vachon ML. Social support networks and the crisis of bereavement. Soc Sci Med 1977;11(1):35-41.

Walker VA, Hoskin PJ, Hanks GW, White ID. Evaluation of WHO Analgesic Guidelines for Cancer Pain in a hospital-based palliative care unit. J Pain Symptom Manage 1988;3(3):145-9.

Wallston K, Wallston B, Smith S, et al. Perceived control and health. Current Psychological Research and Reviews 1987;6(1):5-25.

Walsh TD. Oral morphine in chronic cancer pain. Pain 1984;18:1-11.

Wang BC, Hillman DE, Spielholz NI, Turndorf H. Chronic neurological deficits and nesacaine-CE: an effect of the anesthetic, 2-chloroprocaine, or the antioxidant, sodium bisulfite? Anesth Analg 1984;63:445-7.

Ward SE, Goldberg N, Miller-McCauley V, Mueller C, Nolan A, Pawlik-Plank D, Robbins A, Stormoen D, Weissman DE. Patient-related barriers to management of cancer pain. Pain 1993;52(3):319-24.

Watson CP, Evans RJ. A comparative trial of amitriptyline and zimelidine in post-herpetic neuralgia. Pain 1985;23(4):387-94.

Watson CP, Evans RJ, Reed K, Merskey H, Goldsmith L, Warsh J. Amitriptyline versus placebo in postherpetic neuralgia. Neurology 1982;32:671-3.

Weekes DP, Savedra MC. Adolescent cancer: coping with treatment-related pain. J Pediatr Nurs 1988;3(5):318-28.

Weingart WA, Sorkness CA, Earhart RH. Analgesia with oral narcotics and added ibuprofen in cancer patients. Clin Pharm 1985;4(1):53-8.

Weiss HJ, Aledort LM, Kochwa S. The effect of salicylates on the hemostatic properties of platelets in man. J Clin Invest 1968;47(9):2169-80.

Weissman DE. Glucocorticoid treatment for brain metastases and epidural spinal cord compression: a review. J Clin Oncol 1988;6:543-51.

Weissman DE, Burchman SL, Dinndorf PA, Dahl JL. Handbook of cancer pain management. 2nd ed. Madison, WI: Wisconsin Cancer Pain Initiative; 1988 [updated 1990, 1992].

Weissman DE, Burchman SL, Dinndorf PA, Dahl JL. Handbook of cancer pain management. 3rd ed. Madison, WI: Wisconsin Cancer Pain Initiative; 1992; p. 7-8.

Weissman DE, Haddox JD. Opioid pseudoaddiction—an iatrogenic syndrome. Pain 1989;36(3):363-6.

Weissman DE, Joranson DE, Hopwood MB. Wisconsin physicians' knowledge and attitudes about opioid analgesic regulations. Wis Med J 1991;90(12):671-5.

Wells DG, Bjorksten AR. Monoamine oxidase inhibitors revisited. Can J Anaesth 1989;36(1):67-74.

White JC, Sweet WH. Pain and the neurosurgeon. A forty-year experience. Springfield: Thomas Press; 1969.

Whitney SL. Physical agents: heat and cold modalities. In: Scully R, Barnes M, editors. Physical therapy. Philadelphia: JB Lippincott Co.; 1989. p. 844-75.

Wilkie D, Lovejoy N, Dodd M, Tesler M. Cancer pain control behaviors: description and correlation with pain intensity. Oncol Nurs Forum 1988;15(6):723-31.

Wilner D. Radiology of bone tumors and allied disorders. In: Wilner DM, editor. Cancer metastasis to bone. Philadelphia: WB Saunders; 1982. p. 3641-908.

Wilson JF. Behavioral preparation for surgery: benefit or harm? J Behav Med 1981;4(1):79-102.

Wisconsin Cancer Pain Initiative. Cancer pain can be relieved: a guide for patients and families. Madison, WI: Wisconsin Cancer Pain Initiative; 1988.

Wisconsin Cancer Pain Initiative. Children's cancer pain can be relieved. Madison, WI: Wisconsin Cancer Pain Initiative; 1989.

Wisconsin Cancer Pain Initiative. Jeff asks about cancer pain. Madison, WI: Wisconsin Cancer Pain Initiative; 1990.

World Health Organization. Cancer pain relief and palliative care. Report of a WHO expert committee [World Health Organization Technical Report Series, 804]. Geneva, Switzerland: World Health Organization; 1990. p. 1-75.

Yajnik S, Singh GP, Singh G, Kumar M. Phenytoin as a coanalgesic in cancer pain. J Pain Symptom Manage 1992;7:209-13.

Yaksh TL, Rudy TA. Analgesia mediated by a direct spinal action of narcotics. Science 1976;192(4246):1357-8.

Yanagida H, Suwa K, Trouwborst A, Erdmann W, et al. Electrical stimulation of the pituitary—its use in the treatment of cancer pain. Pain Clinic 1988;2(4):225-8.

Yasco JM, Verfurth M. Closing comment: economic trends. Semin Oncol Nurs 1992;8(2):156-8.

Young RF, Brechner T. Electrical stimulation of the brain for relief of intractable pain due to cancer. Cancer 1986;57(6):1266-72.

Young RJ, Clarke BF. Pain relief in diabetic neuropathy: the effectiveness of imipramine and related drugs. Diabetic Med 1985;2(5):363-6.

Zeltzer LK, Altman A, Cohen D, LeBaron S, Maunuksela EL, Schechter NL. American Academy of Pediatrics Report of the Subcommittee on the Management of Pain Associated with Procedures in Children with Cancer. Pediatrics 1990;86(5):826-31.

Zeltzer LK, Jay SM, Fisher DM. The management of pain associated with pediatric procedures. Pediatr Clin North Am 1989;36(4):941-64.

Zeltzer L, LeBaron S. Hypnosis and nonhypnotic techniques for reduction of pain and anxiety during painful procedures in children and adolescents with cancer. J Pediatr 1982;101(6):1032-5.

Zucker MB, Rothwell KG. Differential influences of salicylate compounds on platelet aggregation and serotonin release. Curr Ther Res 1978;Feb 23(2):194-9.

Acronyms

ACS	American Cancer Society
AHCPR	Agency for Health Care Policy and Research
AIDS	Acquired immunodeficiency syndrome
APAP	Acetaminophen
ARS	Adjective rating scale
AZT	Zidovudine, commonly referred to as AZT
CNS	Central nervous system
CSA	Controlled Substances Act
CSF	Cerebrospinal fluid
CT scan	Computed tomographic scan
EMLA	Eutectic mixture of local anesthetic
FDA	Food and Drug Administration
GI	Gastrointestinal
HIV	Human immunodeficiency virus
MAOI	Monamine oxidase inhibitors
MRI	Magnetic resonance imaging
NRS	Numerical rating scale
NSAID	Nonsteroidal anti-inflammatory drug
PCA	Patient-controlled analgesia
TENS	Transcutaneous electrical nerve stimulation
WHO	World Health Organization
VAS	Visual analogue scale

Glossary

Ablative surgery. Surgical procedures performed on peripheral nerves, the spinal cord, the brain or brain stem that relieve pain by permanent disruption of nerve pathways.

Acupuncture. The piercing of specific body sites with needles to produce pain relief.

Addiction (psychological dependence). Pattern of compulsive drug use characterized by a continued craving for an opioid and the need to use the opioid for effects other than pain relief.

Adjuvant analgesic drug. A drug that is not a primary analgesic but that research has shown to have independent or additive analgesic properties.

Anxiolysis. Sedation or hypnosis used to reduce anxiety, agitation, or tension.

Anxiolytic. Medication used to reduce anxiety, agitation, or tension.

Behavioral techniques. A coping strategy in which patients are taught to monitor and evaluate their own behavior and to modify their reactions to pain.

Biofeedback. A process in which a person learns to influence reliably physiologic responses of two kinds: those that are not ordinarily under voluntary control or those that ordinarily are easily regulated but for which regulation has broken down because of trauma or disease.

Breakthrough pain. Intermittent exacerbations of pain that can occur spontaneously or in relation to specific activity.

Cognitive reappraisal. A coping strategy in which patients are taught to monitor and evaluate negative thoughts and replace them with more positive thoughts and images.

Conscious sedation. "Light sedation" during which the patient retains airway reflexes and responses to verbal stimuli.

Counterstimulation. Application of moderate to intense sensory stimulation, such as with cold, heat, rubbing, pressure, or electrical current, so as to decrease perception of pain at the same or a distant site.

Cryotherapy. The therapeutic use of cold to reduce discomfort; limit progression of tissue edema; or break a cycle of muscle spasm. Cryotherapy is a form of counterirritation.

Deafferentation pain. Pain due to loss of sensory input into the central nervous system, as occurs with avulsion of the brachial plexus or other types of lesions of peripheral nerves or because of pathology of the central nervous system.

Distraction. The cognitive strategy of focusing attention on stimuli other than pain or negative emotions that accompany pain.

Dysesthesia. An unpleasant abnormal sensation, whether spontaneous or evoked.

Epidural. Situated within the spinal canal, on or outside the dura mater (tough membrane surrounding the spinal cord); synonyms are "extradural" and "peridural."

Equianalgesic. Having equal pain-killing effect; morphine sulfate, 10 mg intramuscularly, is generally used for opioid analgesic comparisons.

Horner's syndrome. A Pancoast tumor that involves both the upper and lower brachial plexus.

Hyperpathia. A painful syndrome, characterized by increased reaction to a stimulus, especially a repetitive stimulus, as well as an increased threshold.

Hypnosis. A state of heightened awareness and focused concentration that can be used to manipulate the perception of pain.

Iatrogenic. Induced inadvertently by the medical treatment or procedures of a physician.

Imagery. A cognitive-behavioral strategy that uses mental images as an aid to relaxation.

Incident pain. See "movement-related pain."

Intrathecal. Within a sheath, e.g., cerebrospinal fluid that is contained within the dura mater.

Lancinating. Characterized by piercing or stabbing sensations.

Local nerve block. Infiltration of a local anesthetic around a peripheral nerve so as to produce anesthesia in the area supplied by the nerve.

Mixed opioid agonist-antagonist. A compound that has an affinity for two or more types of opioid receptors and blocks opioid effects on one receptor type while producing opioid effects on a second receptor type.

Movement-related pain. A type of breakthrough pain that is related to specific activity, such as eating, defecation, socializing, or walking. Also referred to as incident pain.

Mucositis. Inflammation of a mucous membrane. Oral mucositis is a common complication of chemotherapy and radiation therapy.

Music therapy. A form of distraction that uses music as an aid to relaxation.

Myofascial pain. A large group of muscle disorders characterized by the presence of hypersensitive points, called trigger points, within one or more muscles and/or the investing connective tissue together with a syndrome of pain, muscle spasm, tenderness, stiffness, limitation of motion, weakness, and occasionally autonomic dysfunction.

Neurolytic block. The injection of a chemical agent to cause destruction and consequent prolonged interruption of peripheral somatic or sympathetic nerves, or in some cases, the neuraxis.

Neuropathic pain. Pain that results from a disturbance of function or pathologic change in a nerve; in one nerve mononeuropathy; in several nerves, mononeuropathy multiplex; if diffuse and bilateral, polyneuropathy.

Nociceptive. The process of pain transmission; usually relating to a receptive neuron for painful sensations.

NSAID. Aspirin-like drug that reduces inflammation (and hence pain) arising from injured tissue.

Opioid agonist. Any morphine-like compound that produces bodily effects including pain relief, sedation, constipation, and respiratory depression.

Opioid partial agonist. A compound that has an affinity for and stimulates physiologic activity at the same cell receptors as opioid agonists but that produces only a partial (i.e., submaximal) bodily response.

Opiate receptor. Opiate-binding sites found throughout primary afferents and the neuraxis.

Pain. An unpleasant sensory and emotional experience associated with actual or potential tissue damage or described in terms of such damage.

Palliative therapy. A procedure such as chemotherapy, radiation therapy, or surgery that is performed to relieve or ease pain.

Pancoast tumor. Tumor originating from the superior sulcus of the lung that invades all or a portion of the brachial plexus.

PCA. Self-administration of analgesics by a patient instructed in doing so; usually refers to self-dosing with intravenous opioid (e.g., morphine) administered by means of a programmable pump.

Physical dependence. Physiologic adaptation of the body to the presence of opioid is required to maintain the same level of analgesia.

Physical modalities. Therapeutic interventions that use physical methods, such as heat, cold, massage, or exercise, to relieve pain.

Progressive muscle relaxation. A cognitive-behavioral strategy in which muscles are alternately tensed and then relaxed in a systematic fashion.

Pseudoaddiction. Pattern of drug-seeking behavior of pain patients receiving inadequate pain management that can be mistaken for addiction.

Psychological dependence (addiction). Pattern of compulsive drug use characterized by a continued craving for an opioid and the need to use the opioid for effects other than pain relief.

Psychosocial intervention. A therapeutic intervention that uses cognitive, cognitive-behavioral, behavioral, and supportive interventions to relieve pain. These include patient education, interventions aimed at aiding relaxation, psychotherapy, and structured or peer support.

Relaxation. A state of relative freedom from both anxiety and skeletal muscle tension.

Self-statement. Involves instructing patients to substitute positive thoughts for such negative ones as "I can't stand this" or "How much longer will this go on?"

Suffering. A state of severe distress associated with events that threaten the intactness of the person.

Tolerance. A common physiologic result of chronic opioid use; it means that a larger dose of opioid is required to maintain the same level of analgesia.

TENS. A method of producing electroanalgesia through electrodes applied to the skin.

Contributors

Cancer Pain Panel Members: Biosketches

Ada K. Jacox, RN, PhD, FAAN, Co-Chair   1991–94
Independence Foundation Chair of Health Policy
School of Nursing
The Johns Hopkins University
Baltimore, Maryland
Specialties: Health Policy, Outcomes Research

Dr. Jacox is a nurse who has had extensive experience in health policy and in the analysis of scientific evidence for application to clinical practice. She has conducted research on pain assessment and has published her work in numerous publications. She serves as editor of the Mosby Year Book of Pain. Her responsibilities as Co-Chair of the panel included overseeing the process of review of scientific evidence and, together with the Co-Chairs, directing the work of the panel, consultants, and staff, in the development, testing, and dissemination of the guidelines.

Daniel B. Carr, MD, Co-Chair   1991–92
Special Consultant 1992–94
Director, Division of Pain Management
Department of Anesthesia
Massachusetts General Hospital
Boston, Massachusetts
Specialties: Anesthesiology, Endocrinology

Dr. Carr has extensive clinical and research experience in pain management. In addition to cochairing the first half of the panel's work, Dr. Carr wrote and edited major sections of the guideline. Dr. Carr is Associate Professor of Anesthesiology and Medicine at Harvard Medical School. He participated in the development of the American Pain Society's quality assurance standards for pain management. Dr. Carr serves on the editorial board of the *Clinical Journal of Pain* and is Editor-in-Chief of *Pain: Clinical Update,* published by the International Association for the Study of Pain. His special interests are stress physiology, analgesic peptides, and burn pain.

Richard Payne, MD, Co-Chair   1992–94
Panel Member 1991–92
Director, Pain and Symptom Management Section
MD Anderson Cancer Center
Houston, Texas
Specialties: Neurology, Oncology

Dr. Payne has done extensive research on opioid analgesic pharmacology in cancer pain and sickle cell pain. He was a member of the Ad Hoc Subcommittee on Medical School Courses and Curricula, International Association for the Study of Pain. He is a member of the Editorial Board of the *Clinical Journal of Pain* and a member of the Board of Directors of the American Pain Society. Dr. Payne's responsibilities as Co-Chair included writing major sections of the guideline and directing the work of the panel.

Charles B. Berde, MD, PhD   1992–94
Director, Pain Treatment Service
Children's Hospital
Boston, Massachusetts
Specialties: Pediatrics, Anesthesia, Critical Care

Dr. Berde is an Associate Professor of Anesthesiology and Pediatrics at Harvard Medical School, the Director of the Pain Treatment Service at the Children's Hospital, and a nationally recognized authority on pain management in children. He has extensive clinical and research experience in pain management and mechanisms of pain and its relief. Dr. Berde is the Scientific Editor of the *International Association for the Study of Pain Newsletter* and is on the Editorial Board of the *American Pain Society Journal.*

William Breitbart, MD   1991–94
Associate Member
Memorial Sloan-Kettering Cancer Center
New York, New York
Specialties: Psychiatry, Internal Medicine

Dr. Breitbart is an Assistant Professor of Psychiatry at Cornell University Medical College, Medical Director of the Memorial Hospital Psychiatry Service Home Care Program, and a nationally recognized authority on psychiatric aspects of cancer pain management. He has written about psychiatric and psychological contributions to symptom management in cancer and AIDS patients. Dr. Breitbart is Co-Chair of the International Association for the Study of Pain's Task Force on Pain in AIDS. He is a founding member of the American Society for Psychiatric Oncology/AIDS and is on the Editorial Board of the *Journal of Pain and Symptom Management.*

Joanna M. Cain, MD   1992–94
Director, Women's Clinic
Division of Gynecologic Oncology
University of Washington Hospital
Seattle, Washington
Specialties: Obstetrics, Gynecologic Oncology

Dr. Cain is a gynecologic oncologist with extensive clinical experience in the management of pain in patients with pelvic malignancy. She is an Associate Professor of Obstetrics and Gynecology at the University of Washington Medical School. She has an interest and expertise in medical ethics and is a member of the Association of Professors of Gynecology and Obstetrics Ethics Committee. She also serves as a consultant on ethical issues to the National Institutes of Health.

C. Richard Chapman, PhD   1991–92
Professor, Department of Anesthesiology
University of Washington School of Medicine
Director, Pain and Toxicity Research Program
Fred Hutchinson Cancer Research Center
Seattle, Washington
Specialty: Psychology

Dr. Chapman is a psychologist who has studied pain since the early 1970's. His research on both experimental and clinical pain has focused on the assessment and treatment of acute and chronic pain, including cancer pain and acupuncture. He brought to the panel an understanding of psychological interventions for pain and opioid analgesia. He is a past member of the Board of Directors of the American Pain Society and Editor of the *Bulletin of the American Pain Society.*

Charles S. Cleeland, PhD   1992–94
Director, Pain Research Group
Professor of Neurology
University of Wisconsin Medical School
Madison, Wisconsin
Specialty: Psychology

Dr. Cleeland is well known for his work documenting the severity and effect of pain due to cancer as well as the variability in cancer pain treatment. Dr. Cleeland is Chair of the United States Cancer Pain Relief Committee and has served as Co-Chair of the National Cancer Institute's Cancer Pain Work Group. He is the Director of the World Health Organization's Collaborating Center for Symptom Evaluation for the cancer unit and has participated in the development of WHO international demonstration projects in cancer pain relief.

Betty R. Ferrell, RN, PhD, FAAN   1991–94
Associate Research Scientist, Nursing Research
City of Hope Medical Center
Duarte, California
Specialties: Oncology, Nursing

Dr. Ferrell has expertise as a researcher and clinician in the management of cancer pain, particularly pain in the elderly patient and pain at home. She has had experience in incorporating pain management into quality assurance programs. Dr. Ferrell's other research interests are in ethical and clinical decisionmaking in cancer pain, quality of life in cancer survivors, and the cost of pain management.

Rebecca S. Finley, PharmD, MS   1992–94
Head, Section of Pharmacy Services
University of Maryland Cancer Center
Associate Professor of Oncology
Associate Professor of Pharmacy Practice
University of Maryland School of Pharmacy
Baltimore, Maryland
Specialty: Institutional Pharmacy

Dr. Finley has expertise as a researcher, clinician, and educator in the management of chemotherapy and pain in cancer patients. She currently serves on the Board of Directors of the American Society of Hospital Pharmacists (ASHP) and is a former Chairperson for the ASHP Special Interest Group on Oncology. She currently chairs the Editorial Advisory Board, Panel on Oncology for the journal *Annals of Pharmacotherapy.*

Nancy O. Hester, RN, PhD, FAAN   1991–94
Associate Professor, School of Nursing
University of Colorado Health Sciences Center
Denver, Colorado
Specialties: Pediatrics, Research Methods

Dr. Hester, a nurse, began studying pain in children in 1975. Her research focuses on the child's perception of pain experiences; comfort for the child in pain; the measurement of procedural, postoperative, and cancer pain in children; nurse clinical decisionmaking about pain in children; and pain assessment and management practices on pediatric units. She was a member of the National Center for Nursing Research's panel to set priorities in the study of pain and currently serves on the Nursing Research Study Section for the National Institutes of Health.

C. Stratton Hill, Jr., MD   1991–92
Professor of Medicine
University of Texas
MD Anderson Cancer Center
Houston, Texas
Specialty: Oncology

Dr. Hill was the Director of MD Anderson's Pain Service for 10 years. His major interest is cultural and societal barriers to adequate pain control when opioids are required. He coauthored a bill, The Intractable Pain Treatment Act, and was instrumental in its passage by the 71st Session of the Texas Legislature in July 1989. Dr. Hill is on the Editorial Board of the *Pain Clinic Journal.*

W. David Leak, MD, FACPM   1992–94
Medical Director, Pain Control Consultants
Westerville, Ohio
Specialty: Pain Medicine

Dr. Leak is an adjutant staff member at the Cleveland Clinic Foundation. His major interests are in the neuroaugmentation of the CNS and the cultural and social aspects of pain management. He serves on the Examination Committee of the American College of Pain Medicine. Dr. Leak is Chairman of the National Medical Association Political Action Committee.

Arthur G. Lipman, PharmD   1991–92
Professor of Clinical Pharmacy
College of Pharmacy
University of Utah
Salt Lake City, Utah
Specialty: Pharmacology in Pain Symptom Control

Dr. Lipman practices in the Pain Management Center at University Hospital, University of Utah. He was a member of the National Cancer Institute Demonstration Project of Hospice Care in New Haven, Connecticut, and is now pharmacologic consultant and a past president of Community Hospice in Utah. His research interests focus on cancer pain management. While on sabbatical leave from the University of Utah, he collaborated in the development of a cancer pain data system at Sir Michael Sobell House, Churchill Hospital, University of Oxford, England. Dr. Lipman serves on the Pain Management Advisory Group of the American Cancer Society and is Editor of the *Journal of Pharmaceutical Care in Pain and Symptom Control.*

Catherine L. Logan   1992–94
Executive Director and Founder, Living Through Cancer, Inc.
Board of Advisors, National Coalition for Cancer Survivorship
Albuquerque, New Mexico
Consumer Representative

Catherine Logan is a 15-year survivor of invasive cervical cancer and the cofounder of the National Coalition for Cancer Survivorship. She served as the first Executive Director of this organization from 1986 to 1991. She is an outspoken advocate for community-based, grassroots cancer support organizations and has given presentations on the survivorship movement at conferences and workshops across the country.

Charles L. McGarvey, PT, MS   1991–92
Chief, Physical Therapy Section
Rehabilitation Medicine Department
Warren G. Magnuson Clinical Center
National Institutes of Health
Bethesda, Maryland
Specialty: Physical Therapy

Mr. McGarvey is a physical therapist and a Commander in the Commissioned Corps of the U.S. Public Health Service. Before coming to the National Institutes of Health in 1983, he was Deputy Chief of the Physical Therapy Department at the U.S. Public Health Service Hospital in Whiteriver, Arizona, and before that a staff physical therapist at the U.S. Public Health Service Hospital in Norfolk, Virginia. He is past President of the Oncology Section of the American Physical Therapy Association and Editor of the text *Physical Therapy for the Cancer Patient.*

Christine A. Miaskowski, RN, PhD, FAAN   1991–92
Associate Professor
Department of Physiological Nursing
University of California, San Francisco
San Francisco, California
Specialty: Oncology

Dr. Miaskowski is an oncology clinical nurse specialist with extensive experience in the development of standards of practice and their monitoring for quality assurance. She served as a member of the American Pain Society committee that developed quality assurance standards for pain management. Her research focuses on mechanisms of opioid-induced analgesia. Dr. Miaskowski is on the Board of Directors of the American Pain Society.

David Stevenson Mulder, MD   1991–92
Professor of Surgery, McGill University
Surgeon-in-Chief, Montreal General Hospital
Montreal, Quebec, Canada
Specialty: Cardiothoracic Surgery

Dr. Mulder is an academic surgeon with a specialty in cardiothoracic surgery. He has authored, among numerous publications, texts on surgical research and acute life support. In 1989, he was Secretary of the International Trauma Society and, in 1990, President of the Canadian Association of Clinical Surgeons.

Judith A. Paice, RN, PhD   1992–94
Clinical Specialist, Pain Management
Neuroscience Institute
Rush-Presbyterian-St. Luke's Medical Center
Chicago, Illinois
Specialties: Neurosurgery, Oncology

Dr. Paice is a nurse who has written and lectured extensively in the area of cancer pain management, including the use of intrathecal morphine infusions for intractable cancer pain. Her research interests are in the physiology of pain transmission and the role of new agents in the treatment of neuropathic pain. She has served on the Editorial Review Board of *Oncology Nursing Forum* and currently serves on the Board of the *Year Book of Oncology Nursing.*

Barbara S. Shapiro, MD   1991–92
Associate Director, Pain Management Program
Children's Hospital of Philadelphia
Assistant Professor of Pediatrics
University of Pennsylvania School of Medicine
Philadelphia, Pennsylvania
Specialties: General Pediatrics, Pain Management

Dr. Shapiro is a general pediatrician with specialty training in pediatric hematology and oncology. She participated in the formation of an interdisciplinary pediatric pain service, and the majority of her clinical and research efforts are in the area of pain assessment and management. She has been particularly active in the areas of sickle cell- and cancer-related pain.

Edward B. Silberstein, MD, FACNP   1992–94
Associate Director, E. L. Saenger Radioisotope Laboratory
University of Cincinnati Medical Center
Professor of Medicine and Radiology
University of Cincinnati College of Medicine
Cincinnati, Ohio
Specialties: Nuclear Medicine, Internal Medicine,
    Hematology, Oncology

Dr. Silberstein is a nuclear medicine physician with extensive experience in the use of radiopharmaceuticals to palliate metastatic cancer
pain. He is a prolific researcher and has published extensively on the
use of radiopharmaceuticals. Dr. Silberstein serves as Consultant for
the United States Pharmacopeia, the Department of Health and
Human Services, the Centers for Disease Control, the Nuclear
Regulatory Commission, and the Department of Energy. He is the
Nuclear Medicine Section Editor of the *Journal of the American
Medical Association.*

Rev. Robert S. Smith, PhD   1991–92
Director, Institute for Medicine in Contemporary Society
State University Medical Center at Stony Brook
Stony Brook, New York
Specialties: Religion, Ethics

Father Smith was ordained to the Roman Catholic priesthood in 1958.
During the past 10 years, he has taught bioethics in the School of
Medicine, State University of New York, Stony Brook, and has served
on numerous state and national boards dealing with medicine and
ethics. He is a member of the New York State Governor's Task Force
on Life and Law and the New York State Cardiac Advisory
Committee; Fr. Smith is on the Board of Directors of the United
Network for Organ Sharing.

Jeanne Stover   1991–92
Cofounder of Living Through Cancer, Inc.
Sandia Park, New Mexico
Consumer Representative

Ms. Stover was a 23-year survivor of metastatic breast cancer who had
experienced cancer pain for many years. She represented the National
Coalition for Cancer Survivorship on the panel. Ms. Stover was
cofounder of the Living Through Cancer Survivorship Center, one of
the country's largest and most active community-based local cancer
support/survivorship organizations. She died in January 1993.

Carole V. Tsou, MD   1991–92
Residency Program Director
University of Hawaii
Department of Family Practice
Mililani, Hawaii
Specialty: Family Medicine

Dr. Tsou is a family physician who has been involved in the education of family physicians at the undergraduate, graduate, and continuing education levels. She completed a research fellowship in family medicine at the University of California, Los Angeles, and formerly was Assistant Director of the Education Division of the American Academy of Family Physicians.

Loretta Vecchiarelli   1991–92
Ludlow, Massachusetts
Consumer Representative

Ms. Vecchiarelli is a rehabilitation counselor and a physician's assistant. She suffered serious burn injuries as an adult and subsequently underwent treatment and rehabilitation, which included experiencing repeated episodes of treatment-induced pain. She has served as a consumer representative on the panel.

David E. Weissman, MD   1992–94
Associate Professor of Medicine
Division of Cancer and Blood Diseases
Medical College of Wisconsin
Milwaukee, Wisconsin
Specialties: Internal Medicine, Oncology

Dr. Weissman has expertise as a clinician, researcher, and educator in cancer pain management. He is the Director of the Cancer Pain Role Model Program—a physician education program—of the Wisconsin Cancer Pain Initiative. He is nationally known for his contributions to cancer pain education and his interest in regulatory barriers to cancer pain relief.

Other Contributors[1]

Consultants

Gerard Anderson, PhD
Associate Professor of
Health Policy and Management
Johns Hopkins University
Baltimore, Maryland

Ehud Arbit, MD
Chief, Neurosurgery Service
Memorial Sloan-Kettering
Cancer Center
New York, New York

Catherine Berkey, DSc, MA
Technology Assessment Group
Harvard University School of
Public Health
Boston, Massachusetts

Andrew P. Brown, MRCP, FRCR
Radiation Oncologist
Elliot Hospital
Manchester, New Hampshire

Thomas C. Chalmers, MD
Technology Assessment Group
Harvard University School of
Public Health
Boston, Massachusetts

June L. Dahl, PhD
Professor of Pharmacology
University of Wisconsin-Madison
Medical School
Madison, Wisconsin

Stuart L. Du Pen, MD
Director,
Pain Management Service
Swedish Tumor Institute
Swedish Medical Center
Seattle, Washington

Hurdis Griffith, RN, PhD, FAAN
Senior Policy Advisor
Office of Disease Prevention
and Health Promotion
U.S. Public Health Service,
Department of Health and
Human Services
Washington, District of Columbia

Stuart A. Grossman, MD
Director, Neuro-Oncology
Associate Professor of Oncology,
Medicine, and Neurosurgery
The Johns Hopkins
Oncology Center
Baltimore, Maryland

Bernard Hammes, PhD
Gundersen Clinic
LaCrosse, Wisconsin

Nora A. Janjan, MD
Associate Professor of Radiation
Oncology
MD Anderson Cancer Center
Houston, Texas

David E. Joranson, MSSW
Associate Director
Pain Research Group
University of Wisconsin-Madison
Medical School
Madison, Wisconsin

E. M. Kolassa, MBA
Research Associate
Research Institute of
Pharmaceutical Sciences
The University of Mississippi
University, Mississippi

---

[1]Being listed in this section does not necessarily imply endorsement of the guideline.

Mathew Lefkowitz, MD
Assistant Professor of
Anesthesiology
Director,
Pain Management Service
State University of New York
Health Science Center at
Brooklyn
Brooklyn, New York

Margo McCaffery, RN,
MS, FAAN
Consultant in the Nursing Care
of Patients with Pain
Los Angeles, California

Patricia A. McGrath, PhD
Director, Child Health
Research Institute
University of Western Ontario
at the Children's Hospital of
Western Ontario
London, Ontario, Canada

Frederick Mosteller, PhD
Professor
Department of Health Policy
and Management
Harvard University School
of Public Health
Boston, Massachusetts

Raphael E. Pollock, MD, PhD
Associate Professor of Surgery
Deputy Chairman, Department
of Surgical Oncology
University of Texas
MD Anderson Cancer Center
Houston, Texas

Robyn Shapiro, JD
Director, Center for the
Study of Bioethics
Medical College of Wisconsin
Milwaukee, Wisconsin

Vivian R. Sheidler, RN, MS
Clinical Nurse Specialist
Johns Hopkins Oncology Center
Baltimore, Maryland

Judith A. Spross, MS, RN,
OCN, FAAN
Oncology Nurse Consultant
Boston, Massachusetts

Sridhar V. Vasudevan, MD
Clinical Professor of Physical
Medicine and Rehabilitation
Medical Director
Pain Rehabilitation Center
Elmbrook Memorial Hospital
Brookfield, Wisconsin

Anna Williams, RN, MN
Clinical Nurse Specialist
Swedish Tumor Institute
Swedish Medical Center
Seattle, Washington

Melissa Wolff, MS, PT
Coordinator
Pain Consultants Network
University of Tennessee
Medical Center
Knoxville, Tennessee

Peer Reviewers

Barbara R. Abela, RNC
Nursing Supervisor
Visiting Nurse Association of
Southeast Michigan
Detroit, Michigan

Robert G. Addison, MD
Director of Medical Planning
Professor,
Clinical Orthopaedic Surgery
Professor,
Clinical Rehabilitation Medicine
Rehabilitation Institute
of Chicago
Chicago, Illinois

Barbara Lewin Allen, MSN
Nursing Supervisor
Visiting Nurse Association
of Southeast Michigan
Oak Park, Michigan

John Ambre, MD, PhD
Director, Toxicology and
Drug Abuse
American Medical Association
Chicago, Illinois

Paul N. Anderson, MD
Founder, Director
Cancer Center of
Colorado Springs
Colorado Springs, Colorado

Gerald M. Aronoff, MD
Director, Boston Pain Center
Assistant Clinical Professor
Tufts Medical School
Melrose, Massachusetts

Michael A. Ashburn, MD
Director, Acute Pain Service
Assistant Professor of
Anesthesiology
University of Utah
Health Science Center
Salt Lake City, Utah

James Atkins, MD
Oncologist
North Carolina Pain Initiative
Goldsboro, North Carolina

Carol Balmer, PharmD
Associate Professor
University of Colorado
School of Pharmacy
Denver, Colorado

Anne E. Belcher, PhD
Associate Professor and Chair
University of Maryland,
School of Nursing
Baltimore, Maryland

Miles J. Belgrade, MD
Director, Hennepin Pain Clinic
Department of Neurology
Hennepin County
Medical Center
Minneapolis, Minnesota

Elizabeth Benson, RN
Hospice Nursing Coordinator
Lutheran Hospice Care
Wheat Ridge, Colorado

J. Andrew Billings, MD
Assistant Clinical Professor
of Medicine
Harvard Medical School
Associate Physician
Massachusetts General Hospital
Boston, Massachusetts

Diane Blum, MSW
Executive Director
Cancer Care, Inc.
New York, New York

Albert L. Blumberg, MD
Vice-Chairman
Department of
Radiation Oncology
Greater Baltimore
Medical Center
Baltimore, Maryland

Nancy L. Bohnet, RN,
MN, FAAN
President/CEO
Home Health Services
Foundation, Inc.
Butler, Pennsylvania

John D. Bonnet, MD
Scott & White Clinic
Temple, Texas

Philip O. Bridenbaugh, MD
Professor and Chairman
Department of Anesthesiology
University of Cincinnati
Medical Center
Cincinnati, Ohio

Dorothy Y. Brockopp, RN, PhD
Nurse Researcher
Associate Professor of Nursing
University of Kentucky
Lexington, Kentucky

Marion E. Broome, RN, PhD
Professor and Assistant
Chairperson
Maternal-Child Nursing
Rush-Presbyterian-St. Luke's
Medical Center
Chicago, Illinois

Beverly A. Buck, RT
Education and Development
Coordinator
Joint Center for
Radiation Therapy
Harvard Medical School
Boston, Massachusetts

James N. Campbell, MD
Associate Director
Department of Neurosurgery
Professor of Neurosurgery
Johns Hopkins University
Medical School
Baltimore, Maryland

Hugh Chaplin, Jr., MD
Emeritus Professor of
Medicine and Pathology
Hospice Volunteer
Washington University
Medical Center
St. Louis, Missouri

Peggy Christ, RN, ET, CIC
Nurse Epidemiologist/
Enterostomal Therapist
Jennie Edmundson Hospital
Council Bluffs, Iowa

David E. Cohen, MD
Director,
Pain Management Program
Children's Hospital
of Philadelphia
Philadelphia, Pennsylvania

Kathleen Colburn, MA
Executive Director
Hospice of Central Iowa
Des Moines, Iowa

B. Eliot Cole, MD
Medical Director, Senior Care
Harris Hospital
Newport, Arkansas

Joseph C. Conger, RPH
Pharmacist
Consultant Pharmacy
Flint, Michigan

Laurel Archer Copp, PhD, DHL
Professor
University of North Carolina
Chapel Hill, North Carolina

Charles J. Coté, MD
Associate Professor
of Anaesthesia
Harvard Medical School
Massachusetts General Hospital
Boston, Massachusetts

Nessa Coyle, RN, MS
Director,
Supportive Care Program
Department of Neurology
Pain Service
Memorial Sloan-Kettering
Cancer Center
New York, New York

Patrick J. Coyne, RN, CS, MSN
Nursing Pain Control Consultant
Medical College of
Virginia Hospitals
Richmond, Virginia

Carol P. Curtiss, RN, MSN, OCN
Oncology Manager/Consultant
Franklin Medical Center
Greenfield, Massachusetts

Lynn Czarniecki, RN, MSN
Children's Hospital
AIDS Program
Newark, New Jersey

June L. Dahl, PhD
Professor of Pharmacology
University of Wisconsin-Madison
Medical School
Madison, Wisconsin

JoAnn Dalton, RN, EdD
Associate Professor
University of North Carolina
at Chapel Hill
School of Nursing
Chapel Hill, North Carolina

Ann L. Daum, RN, MS, CS
Psychiatric Liaison Nurse
Clinical Specialist
Departments of Nursing
and Psychiatry
Rhode Island Hospital
Providence, Rhode Island

Judy M. Diekmann, RN,
DEd, OCN
Associate Professor
Chair, Health Restoration
University of
Wisconsin-Milwaukee
School of Nursing
Milwaukee, Wisconsin

William R. Dinwoodie, MD
Associate Professor of Medicine
H. Lee Moffitt Cancer Center
University of South Florida
Tampa, Florida

Marion B. Dolan, RN
President
Heritage Home Health
Merideth, New Hampshire

Marilee Donovan, RN, PhD
Associate Hospital Director
Oregon Health Sciences University
Portland, Oregon

Mary Jo Dropkin, RN, MSN
Clinical Nurse Specialist
Head and Neck Service
Memorial Sloan-Kettering
Cancer Center
New York, New York

Jeffrey J. Eckardt, MD
Professor of Surgery
and Orthopaedics
University of California,
Los Angeles
Center for Health Sciences
Los Angeles, California

W. Thomas Edwards, PhD, MD
Associate Professor of
Anesthesiology
Director, Pain Relief Service
University of Washington
Harborview Medical Center
Seattle, Washington

Joann M. Eland, RN, PhD,
NAP, FAAN
Associate Professor of Nursing
University of Iowa
Iowa City, Iowa

Thomas E. Elliott, MD
Director of Education and
Research
Duluth Clinic
Duluth, Minnesota

Neil M. Ellison, MD
Associate, Medical Oncology
Geisinger Medical Center
Danville, Pennsylvania

Joyce M. Engel, PhD, OTR
Assistant Professor of
Occupational Therapy
University of Wisconsin-Madison
Madison, Wisconsin

Serdar Erdine
Professor, Chairman
Department of Algology
Medical Faculty of
Istanbul University
Istanbul, Turkey

James Erickson III, MD
Professor of Clinical Anesthesia
Northwestern University
Chicago, Illinois

Margaret Faut-Callahan
DNSc, CRNA, FAAN
Professor
Rush University
College of Nursing
Chicago, Illinois

Fawzy I. Fawzy, MD
Professor, Deputy Chairman
University of California,
Los Angeles
School of Medicine
Los Angeles, California

Phoebe A. Fernald, RN,
MS, OCN
Clinical Nurse
Specialist-Oncology
Rhode Island Hospital
Providence, Rhode Island

F. Michael Ferrante, MD
Director, Pain Treatment Center
Department of Anesthesia
Brigham and Women's Hospital
Boston, Massachusetts

Walter B. Forman, MD, FACP
Associate Chief of Staff
Geriatrics/Extended Care Service
Associate Professor
Medicine, Geriatrics
VA Medical Center
Albuquerque, New Mexico

Michael E. Frederich, MD
Medical Director
Hospice of Southern Illinois, Inc.
Belleville, Illinois

Marvin Frederickson, MD
Medical Oncology Section
Medical Director of Group
Health Hospice Program
Group Health Cooperative of
Puget Sound
Seattle, Washington

Robert W. Frelick, MD, FACP
Consultant, Chronic Disease
Control and Prevention
Delaware Division of
Public Health
Wilmington, Delaware

Rollin M. Gallagher, MD
Director, The Pain Center
Associate Professor,
Psychiatry
State University of New York at
Stony Brook
Stony Brook, New York

Richard Gannon, PharmD
Director of Pharmacy
Pain Control
Hartford Hospital
Hartford, Connecticut

Fannie Gaston-Johansson,
DMSc, RN, FAAN
Director of Post-Masters Program
Associate Professor
Elsie M. Lawler Chair
Johns Hopkins University
Baltimore, Maryland

Madeline E. Gerken, MD
Staff Oncologist
VA Medical Center
Medical Director
Home Health and Hospice Care
Nashua, New Hampshire

Myra Glajchen, DSW
Assistant Director
Cancer Care, Inc.
New York, New York

Gilbert R. Gonzales, MD
Senior Associate Consultant
Mayo Clinic Scottsdale
Scottsdale, Arizona

Lee Green, MD, MPH
Assistant Professor
Department of Family Practice
University of Michigan
Ann Arbor, Michigan

Donna B. Greenberg, MD
Associate Psychiatrist
Assistant Professor Psychiatry
Massachusetts General
Hospital/Harvard Medical School
Boston, Massachusetts

Wendy Gilbert Gronbeck,
RN, OCN, MA
Nurse Clinician
University of Iowa Hospitals
and Clinics
Iowa City, Iowa

Stuart A. Grossman, MD
Director, Neuro-Oncology
Associate Professor of Oncology,
Medicine, and Neurosurgery
The Johns Hopkins
Oncology Center
Baltimore, Maryland

Stephen A. Gudas, PT, PhD
Assistant Professor
Departments of Rehabilitation,
Medicine, and Anatomy
Medical College of Virginia
Richmond, Virginia

Stephen Pernice Gullo, PhD
Director, Health Policies
and Planning
American Institute for Life
Threatening Illness and Loss
Columbia-Presbyterian
Medical Center
New York, New York

Susan Jane Hagan, BSN,
MS, ARNP
Coordinator—Pain Programs
James A. Haley
Veterans Hospital
Tampa, Florida

Gerald E. Hanks, MD
Chairman
Department of Radiation Therapy
Professor of Radiation Therapy
Fox Chase Cancer Center
Philadelphia, Pennsylvania

Kenneth M. Hargreaves,
DDS, PhD
Associate Professor of
Endodontics and Pharmacology
University of Minnesota
School of Dentistry
Minneapolis, Minnesota

Edward P. Hargus, MD
Director of
Pain Management Services
Lawrence and Memorial Hospital
New London, Connecticut

William N. Harsha, MD, MS, JD
President and Board of Advisors
American Academy of
Pain Management
Oklahoma Spine/Pain Clinic
Oklahoma City, Oklahoma

Samuel J. Hassenbusch, MD, PhD
Associate Professor
Neurosurgery
MD Anderson Cancer Center
Houston, Texas

Laura J. Hilderley, RN, MS
Clinical Nurse Specialist
Radiation Oncology
Warwick, Rhode Island

Reginald Ho, MD
Chief, Department of Oncology
and Hematology
Straub Clinic and Hospital
Honolulu, Hawaii

Marilyn Hockenberry-Eaton,
PhD, RN-CS, PNP
Associate Professor
Emory University
Atlanta, Georgia

Jimmie Holland, MD
Chief, Psychiatry Service
Memorial Sloan-Kettering
Cancer Center
New York, New York

Victor J. Hruby, PhD
Regents Professor
Department of Chemistry
University of Arizona
Tucson, Arizona

Jean M. Huls, RN, BSN
Director of Nursing
Hospice of the Valley
Phoenix, Arizona

Terri L. Imada, RN, MS
Oncology Clinical Nurse Specialist
Kuakini Medical Center
Honolulu, Hawaii

Nora A. Janjan, MD
Associate Professor of
Radiation Oncology
MD Anderson Cancer Center
Houston, Texas

David E. Joranson, MSSW
Associate Director
Pain Research Group
University of Wisconsin-Madison
Medical School
Madison, Wisconsin

C. Celeste Johnston, RN, DEd
Associate Professor
McGill University
Montreal, Quebec, Canada

Maryalice Jordan-Marsh, RN, PhD
Director of Nursing
Research Division
Harbor-University of California,
Los Angeles, Medical Center
Torrance, California

A. Robert Kagan, MD
Chief, Radiation Oncology
Southern California Kaiser
Permanente Medical Group
Los Angeles, California

Wayne Katon, MD
Professor of Psychiatry
Department of Psychiatry and
Behavioral Sciences
University of Washington
Medical School
Seattle, Washington

Pamela L. Kedziera, RN,
MSN, OCN
Clinical Manager—
Pain Management Center
Fox Chase Cancer Center
Philadelphia, Pennsylvania

John F. Kerege, PharmD
Clinical Specialist-Oncology
Oregon Health Sciences University
Portland, Oregon

Steven A. King, MD, MS
Associate Director, Pain Center
Associate Professor
Department of Psychiatry and
Human Behavior
Jefferson Medical College
Jefferson Pain Center
Philadelphia, Pennsylvania

Barry M. Kinzbrunner, MD, FACP
Vice President, Clinical Services
Vitas Healthcare Corporation
Miami, Florida

Linda U. Krebs, RN, MS, OCN
Nursing Oncology
Program Leader
University of Colorado
Cancer Center
Denver, Colorado

Stacie E. Krick, PharmD
Assistant Professor of
Pharmacy Practice
Campbell University
School of Pharmacy
Buies Creek, North Carolina

Austin H. Kutscher, DDS
Professor of Dentistry
(in Psychiatry)
College of Physicians
and Surgeons
Columbia University
New York, New York

Robert R. Kutzner, MD
Director
Indiana Pain Institute
Bedford, Indiana

Jacqueline A. LaPerriere, RPh
Pain Service Coordinator
H. Lee Moffitt Cancer Center
Tampa, Florida

Allen Lebovits, PhD
Clinical Associate Professor
Department of Anesthesiology
State University of New York
Health Science Center
at Brooklyn
Brooklyn, New York

Mathew H. M. Lee, MD,
MPH, FACP
Professor and Acting Chairman
Department of Rehabilitation
Medicine
New York University
Medical Center
New York, New York

Mathew Lefkowitz, MD
Assistant Professor of
Anesthesiology
Director,
Pain Management Service
State University of New York
Health Science Center
at Brooklyn
Brooklyn, New York

Mark J. Lema, MD, PhD
Chairman, Department of
Anesthesiology
Roswell Park Cancer Institute
Buffalo, New York

Michael H. Levy, MD, PhD
Co-Director,
Pain Management Center
Fox Chase Cancer Center
Philadelphia, Pennsylvania

Leonard Lichtblau, PhD
Assistant Professor
Department of Pharmacology
University of Minnesota
Minneapolis, Minnesota

Keith D. Lillemoe, MD
Associate Professor of Surgery
Johns Hopkins University
School of Medicine
Baltimore, Maryland

Philipp M. Lippe, MD, FACS,
FACPM
Clinical Associate Professor of
Neurosurgery
Stanford University
San Jose, California

The Rev. Jerry L. Loch,
CRNA, PhD
Pain Management Service
Kishwaukee Hospital
DeKalb, Illinois

John D. Loeser, MD
Professor, Neurological Surgery
and Anesthesiology
University of Washington
Pain Center
Seattle, Washington

David R. Longmire, MD, ABEN
Adjunct Staff, Pain Management
Center
Department of General
Anesthesiology
Division of Research
Anesthesiology
Cleveland Clinic Foundation
Cleveland, Ohio

Neil MacDonald, MD, FRCP(C)
Professor, Palliative Medicine
University of Alberta
Edmonton, Alberta, Canada

Janice Mathews, RN, MEd, MA
Pain Management Specialist
Heritage Home Health
Meredith, New Hampshire

Mitchell B. Max, MD
Chief, Clinical Trials Unit
Neurobiology and
Anesthesiology Branch
National Institute of
Dental Research
National Institutes of Health
Bethesda, Maryland

Margo McCaffery, RN,
MS, FAAN
Consultant in the Nursing Care
of Patients with Pain
Los Angeles, California

Ruth McCorkle, RN, PhD,
FAAN
Professor
School of Nursing
University of Pennsylvania
Philadelphia, Pennsylvania

Francis J. McDonnell, MD,
FFARCSI
Assistant Professor of
Anesthesiology
University of Kentucky
Lexington, Kentucky

Patrick J. McGrath, PhD
Professor
Department of Psychology
Dalhousie University
Halifax, Nova Scotia, Canada

Deborah B. McGuire, RN,
PhD, FAAN
Edith F. Honeycutt Chair
in Oncology Nursing
Associate Professor of Nursing
Nell Hodgson Woodruff
School of Nursing
Emory University
Atlanta, Georgia

Susan C. McMillan, PhD, RN
American Cancer Society
Professor of Oncology Nursing
University of South Florida
College of Nursing
Tampa, Florida

Faye McNaull, RN, CS,
MPH, MBA
Nursing Director
Kansas University Cancer Center
Kansas City, Kansas

Ronald Melzack, PhD
E. P. Taylor Professor
Department of Psychology
McGill University
Montreal, Quebec, Canada

Susan Michlovitz, MS, PT
Adjunct Associate Professor
Hahnemann University
Programs in Physical Therapy
Philadelphia, Pennsylvania

Bonnie L. Minter, RN, MS
Pediatric Hospice Nurse
Massachusetts Cancer
Pain Initiative
Boston, Massachusetts

Jean B. Moen, RN, MS
Senior Vice-President,
Operations
American Cancer Society
Georgia Division
Atlanta, Georgia

Michael F. Mulroy, MD
Staff Anesthesiologist
Department of Anesthesiology
Virginia Mason Medical Center
Seattle, Washington

Maryann R. Nalley, BS, RN
Director of Professional
Education
American Cancer Society
Missouri Division
Jefferson City, Missouri

John Neville, MD
Medical Director
Vesper Society Hospice
San Leandro, California

Lorenz K. Y. Ng, MD
Director, Chronic Pain Program
National Rehabilitation Hospital
Washington, District of Columbia

Doris G. Nuttelman, RN, EdD
Executive Director
New Hampshire Board
of Nursing
Concord, New Hampshire

Donna O'Shaughnessy, RN, OCN
Director
Saint James Hospice
Pontiac, Illinois

James M. Oleske, MD, MPH
Francois-Xavier Bagnoud
Professor of Pediatrics
New Jersey Medical School
Newark, New Jersey

Paul M. Paris, MD, FACEP
Associate Professor and Chief
Division of Emergency Medicine
University of Pittsburgh
School of Medicine
Pittsburgh, Pennsylvania

Steven D. Passik, PhD
Clinical Assistant
Attending Psychologist
Memorial Sloan-Kettering
Cancer Center
New York, New York

Richard B. Patt, MD
Associate Professor
Anesthesiology, Psychiatry,
and Oncology
University of Rochester
School of Medicine and Dentistry
Rochester, New York

David C. Pederson, CRNA
C. R. Nurse Anesthetist
American Association of
Nurse Anesthetists
Carroll, Iowa

Linda K. Person, BSN
Nursing Supervisor, Oncology
Kaiser Foundation Hospital
Honolulu, Hawaii

Jack Pinsky, MD
Associate Clinical Professor
Director, Pain Medicine
University of California, Irvine,
College of Medicine
Orange, California

Russell K. Portenoy, MD
Director of Analgesic Studies,
Pain Service
Memorial Sloan-Kettering
Cancer Center
New York, New York

P. Prithvi Raj, MD
Medical Director
The National Pain Institute
of Georgia
Clinical Professor of
Anesthesiology
The Medical College of Georgia
Atlanta, Georgia

David W. Rattner, MD, FACS
Associate Professor of Surgery
Harvard Medical School
Boston, Massachusetts

L. Brian Ready, MD, FRCP(C)
Professor of Anesthesiology
Director, Acute Pain Service
University of Washington
Medical Center
Seattle, Washington

Marjorie Ream, RN, MN, OCN
Vice President
Hospice Services, Inc.
Butler, Pennsylvania

Patrick M. Renfro, RN, MS, CRC
Rehabilitation Nurse/Counselor
Renfro & Associates
Littleton, Colorado

Linda Jo Rice, MD
Director of Anesthesia Research
Hartford Hospital and
Newington Children's Hospital
Hartford, Connecticut

Anthony J. Richtsmeier, MD
Director, Section of
Behavioral Pediatrics
Rush-Presbyterian-St. Luke's
Medical Center
Chicago, Illinois

Margaret E. Rinehart, MS, PT
Assistant Professor
Thomas Jefferson University
Philadelphia, Pennsylvania

Patricia L. Roberts, MD
Staff Surgeon
Department of
Colon-Rectal Surgery
Lahey Clinic
Burlington, Massachusetts

Susan Howell Robinson, RN,
MS, OCN
Oncology Clinical Nurse Specialist
Massey Cancer Center
Medical College of Virginia
Richmond, Virginia

Michael G. Rock, MD
Associate Professor of
Orthopedic Surgery
Mayo Clinic
Rochester, Minnesota

John Rogers, MD, MPH
Associate Professor of
Family Medicine
Baylor College of Medicine
Houston, Texas

Charles Rosenbaum, MD
Director, Oncology Clinic
Assistant Medical Director
Marlborough Hospital
Marlborough, Massachusetts

Hubert L. Rosomoff, MD,
DMedSc
Professor and Chairman
Department of
Neurological Surgery
University of Miami
Medical Director
Comprehensive Pain and
Rehabilitation Center
Miami, Florida

David A. Rothenberger, MD
Clinical Professor and Chief
Division of
Colon and Rectal Surgery
Department of Surgery
University of Minnesota
St. Paul, Minnesota

B. W. Ruffner, Jr., MD, FACP
Practicing Medical Oncologist
Baronness Erlanger Hospital
Chattanooga, Tennessee

Patricia Rushton, RN, PhD
Oncology Clinical Specialist
VA Medical Center
Salt Lake City, Utah

Paula Sallmén, RN, BAN, OCN
Program Director
Virginia Piper Cancer Institute
Abbott Northwestern Hospital
Minneapolis, Minnesota

Marilyn C. Savedra, RN, DNS, FAAN
Professor and Acting Chair
University of California, San Francisco
School of Nursing
Department of Family Health Care Nursing
San Francisco, California

Neil L. Schechter, MD
Professor of Pediatrics
University of Connecticut
Department of Pediatrics
St. Francis Hospital and Medical Center
Hartford, Connecticut

Betty L. Schmoll, RN, MS
President and CEO
Hospice of Dayton, Inc.
Dayton, Ohio

Florence Seelig, RN, OCN
Oregon Health Sciences University
Portland, Oregon

Mary S. Sheridan, PhD, ACSW
Director of Social Services
Pali Momi Medical Center
Aiea, Hawaii

Andrew G. Shetter, MD, FACP
Chief, Section of Functional and Sterotactic Neurosurgery
Barrow Neurological Institute
Phoenix, Arizona

Mary A. Simmonds, MD
Clinical Assistant Professor of Medicine
Milton S. Hershey Medical Center
Camp Hill, Pennsylvania

Marybeth Singer, RN, BSN, OCN
Nursing Supervisor
Dana Farber Cancer Institute
Boston, Massachusetts

Albert L. Siu, MD, MSPH
Assistant Professor
University of California, Los Angeles
Department of Medicine
Los Angeles, California

Thomas J. Smith, MD, FACP
Assistant Professor of Medicine and Health Administration
Massey Cancer Center
Medical College of Virginia
Richmond, Virginia

William J. Spanos, Jr., MD, FACR
Professor and Vice Chairman
Department of Radiation Oncology
University of Louisville
School of Medicine
James Graham Brown Cancer Center
Louisville, Kentucky

Judith A. Spross, MS, RN, OCN, FAAN
Oncology Nurse Consultant
Boston, Massachusetts

Michael D'Arcy Stanton-Hicks, MB, DrMed, FFARCS
Director,
Pain Management Center
Cleveland Clinic Foundation
Cleveland, Ohio

Alan D. Steinfeld, MD, FACR
Associate Professor of Radiology
New York University
Medical Center
New York, New York

Porter Storey, MD
Medical Director
The Hospice at the
Texas Medical School
Houston, Texas

Carol J. Swenson, RN, MS, OCN
Oncology Clinical Nurse Specialist
Swedish American Hospital
Rockford, Illinois

Karen L. Syrjala, PhD
Psychological Services Director
Pain & Toxicity Program
Fred Hutchinson Cancer
Research Center
Seattle, Washington

Dennis C. Turk, PhD
Professor, Psychiatry,
Anesthesiology &
Behavioral Science
University of Pittsburgh
School of Medicine
Pain Evaluation and
Treatment Institute
Pittsburgh, Pennsylvania

Claudette Varricchio, RN, DSN,
OCN, FAAN
Program Director/
Nurse Consultant
National Cancer Institute
Bethesda, Maryland

Sridhar V. Vasudevan, MD
Clinical Professor of Physical
Medicine and Rehabilitation
Medical Director
Pain Rehabilitation Center
Elmbrook Memorial Hospital
Brookfield, Wisconsin

Sandra Ward, RN, PhD
Assistant Professor
University of Wisconsin-Madison
School of Nursing
Madison, Wisconsin

Carol A. Warfield, MD
Assistant Professor of Anesthesia
Harvard Medical School
Director,
Pain Management Center
Beth Israel Hospital
Boston, Massachusetts

Andrew L. Warshaw, MD
Harold and Ellen Danser
Professor of Surgery
Harvard Medical School
Chief of General Surgery
Massachusetts General Hospital
Boston, Massachusetts

Stuart Weiner, DO
President
Michigan Cancer Pain Initiative
Flint, Michigan

James Whitsitt, MSW
Social Worker
University of Iowa Hospitals
and Clinics
Iowa City, Iowa

Rudolph M. Widmark, MD, PhD
Medical Officer
Food and Drug Administration,
CDER
Rockville, Maryland

Elaine R. Williams, RN, MSW
Regional Director
Instructor
Visiting Nurse Association/
Southeast Michigan
Detroit, Michigan

Melissa Wolff, MS, PT
Coordinator,
Pain Consultants Network
University of Tennessee
Medical Center
Knoxville, Tennessee

Barbara Ann Wright, RPh
Pharmacist
Mid-America Cancer Center
St. John's Regional
Health Center
Springfield, Missouri

Geri Doran Yanes, MD
Assistant Clinical Lecturer
Department of
Radiation Oncology
University of Arizona
Health Sciences Center
Tucson, Arizona

Donald M. Yealy, MD, FACEP
Assistant Professor
Department of
Emergency Medicine
Texas A&M University
Health Sciences Center
Temple, Texas

Lonnie Zeltzer, MD
Professor of Pediatrics
Director, University of
California, Los Angeles
Pediatric Pain Program
Departments of Anesthesiology
and Pediatrics
University of California,
Los Angeles
School of Medicine
Los Angeles, California

List of Site Testers

Anne E. Belcher, PhD
Associate Professor and Chair
University of Maryland
School of Nursing
Baltimore, Maryland

JoAnn Dalton, RN, EdD
Associate Professor
University of North Carolina
at Chapel Hill,
School of Nursing
Chapel Hill, North Carolina

Marion B. Dolan, RN
President
Heritage Home Health
Merideth, New Hampshire

Marilee Donovan, RN, PhD
Associate Hospital Director
Oregon Health Sciences
University
Portland, Oregon

Thomas E. Elliott, MD
Director of
Education and Research
Duluth Clinic
Duluth, Minnesota

Walter B. Forman, MD, FACP
Associate Chief of Staff
Geriatrics/Extended Care Service
Associate Professor,
Medicine, Geriatrics
VA Medical Center
Albuquerque, New Mexico

Marvin Frederickson, MD
Medical Oncology Section
Medical Director of
Group Health Hospice Program
Group Health Cooperative of
Puget Sound
Seattle, Washington

Stephen A. Gudas, PT, PhD
Assistant Professor
Departments of Rehabilitation
Medicine and Anatomy
Medical College of Virginia
Richmond, Virginia

Linda U. Krebs, RN, MS, OCN
Nursing Oncology
Program Leader
University of Colorado
Cancer Center
Denver, Colorado

Jacqueline A. LaPerriere, RPh
Pain Service Coordinator
H. Lee Moffitt Cancer Center
Tampa, Florida

Michael H. Levy, MD, PhD
Co-Director,
Pain Management Center
Fox Chase Cancer Center
Philadelphia, Pennsylvania

Jean B. Moen, RN, MS
Senior Vice-President,
Operations
American Cancer Society
Georgia Division
Atlanta, Georgia

Maryann R. Nalley, BS, RN
Director of Professional
Education
American Cancer Society
Missouri Division
Jefferson City, Missouri

David C. Pederson, CRNA
American Association of Nurse
Anesthetists
Carroll, Iowa

Jeaneva Reese, BA
Staff Assistant, Nursing
Research Division
Harbor-University of California,
Los Angeles, Medical Center
Torrance, California

Patrick M. Renfro, RN, MS, CRC
Rehabilitation Nurse/Counselor
Renfro & Associates
Littleton, Colorado

Organizations and Individuals Providing Additional Scientific, Technical, and Administrative Support:

Johns Hopkins University
Baltimore, Maryland

Janice Fitzgerald Ulmer, RN, PhD, Project Manager
Donna Mahrenholz, RN, PhD,
Dorothy Herron, RN, MSN
Joyce S. Willens, RN, MSN
Yeonghee Shin, PhD
Patricia Stephens, PhD
Leslie C. Dunham, BA

Harvard University
Massachusetts General Hospital
Boston, Massachusetts

Jane Ballantyne, MB, BS
Elon Eisenberg, MD
Evelyn Hall

University of Texas
MD Anderson Cancer Center

Guadalupe Palos, MSW, RN, OCN, CSW

Agency for Health Care Policy and Research
Rockville, Maryland

Kathleen McCormick, PhD, RN
Carole Hudgings, RN, PhD
Margaret Coopey, RN, MS
Karen Carp
Randie Siegel

EEI
Alexandria, Virginia

Martha Sencindiver

Mikalix and Company
Waltham, Massachusetts

Sharon Sokoloff

Other individuals

Valerie Exar
Marsha Whitson

217

Attachment A.

Tables of Scientific Evidence

A1. Scientific evidence for pain reduction in adults

A2. Scientific evidence for pain reduction in children

Explanation of Table of Evidence

The following tables summarize the scientific evidence for interventions to manage pain. The evidence is classified by type and strength. The type of evidence for recommendations is ordinally ranked in categories from I to V. I is evidence from metaanalysis of multiple, well-designed controlled studies. II through V are evidence obtained from experimental studies (II) through case reports and clinical examples (V). Evidence is further subdivided according to whether the studies were conducted on patients with cancer or on other clinical populations. The column in the table labeled "Type of Evidence" summarizes the types of evidence that support interventions discussed in the guideline. The strength and consistency of evidence are described in the text.

Briefly, the strength and consistency of evidence for recommendations summarize the evidence and note whether the evidence is generally consistent or inconsistent. Strength of evidence ranges from A, which is the strongest evidence, to D, which indicates that there is little or no evidence or evidence of type V only. The strength of recommendation is summarized in the column of the tabled labeled "Strength and Consistency of Evidence."

When the strength of evidence is A or B, the panel's recommendations are based primarily on the evidence. When the strength of recommendation is C or D, the panel used the available empirical evidence but based their recommendations primarily on expert judgment. The term "panel consensus" is used when the recommendation is a statement of panel opinion regarding desirable practice and there is evidence that the practice is not commonly being followed.

Two tables are provided. Table A1 summarizes the scientific evidence for the management of pain in adult populations. Table A2 summarizes the scientific evidence for the management of pain in children and adolescents.

A1. Scientific evidence for pain reduction in adults

Intervention		Type of evidence		Strength and consistency of evidence
		Cancer patients	Other patients	
Pharmacologic interventions				
Acetaminophen and NSAIDs	Oral (alone)	Ia	Ib	A
	Oral (adjunct to opioid)	IIa	Ib	A
	Rectal		IIb, IIIb	B
	Parenteral (ketorolac)	Ia	Ib	A
Opioids	Oral	Ia	Ib	A
	Controlled release	Ia		A
	Rectal	IIIa, IVa	IIb	B
	Transdermal	IIIa, Va	IIb	B
	Intramuscular (IM)	IIa	Ib	A
	Subcutaneous (SC)	IIa	Ib	A
	Intravenous (IV)	IIa	Ib	A
	PCA (IV and SC)	Ia	Ib	A
	Epidural and intrathecal	IIa, IIIa	Ib, IIIb	A
	Intracerebral ventricular	IIa, IIIa, IVa		A
Local anesthetics	Oral			
	Topical	IIa		B
	Systemic		IIb	B
	Intravenous	IVa		C
	Epidural and intrathecal	IVa	Ib	A
	Interpleural	Va	IIb, IIIb, Vb	B
Inhalent analgesia	Nitrous oxide	Va	IIb, IIIb	C
Adjuvant analgesics	Corticosteroids	IIa	IIb, IIIb, IVb	B
	Anticonvulsant agents	IIIa	IIb, IIIb, IVb	B
	Antidepressants	IIa, IIIa	Ib, IIb, IIIb, IVb	A
	Neuroleptics	IIa	IIb	C
	Hydroxyzine	IIIa	IIb	C
	Psychostimulants	IIa, Va	IIb	D
	Calcitonin	IIa, IIIa, Va		C
	Bisphosphonates	IIa, IIIa		C
Nonpharmacologic interventions: invasive				
Surgery	Excision or debulking of primary tumor or metastasis	IIIa, Va		D
Neurosurgery	Peripheral neurectomy	Va		D
	Dorsal rhizotomy	IVa, Va		B
	Comissural myelotomy or cordotomy	IVa, Va		B
	Hypophysectomy	IVa, Va		B

Intervention		Type of evidence		Strength and consistency of evidence
		Cancer patients	Other patients	
Nonpharmacologic interventions: invasive (continued)				
Neuroaugmentation	Deep brain stimulation	IVa, Va		B
	Spinal cord stimulation	IVa, Va		C
Neurolytic blocks	Celiac	IIa,IIIa,IVa	IIIb,IVb	A
	Hypogastric	IVa, Va		B
	Intratheca	IIIa, Va		B
	Epidural	Va		D
	Trigeminal	Va	IVb, Vb	B
	Peripheral intercostal	Va		D
Radiotherapy	Local field	IIa		B
	Wide field	IIa		B
	Fractionation: Single dose	IIa		B
	Multidose	IIa		B
	Brachytherapy	IIIa		B
	β-emitting radiopharmaceuticals	Ia, IIa, IIIa		A
Psychosocial	Education: Pain management	IIa, IIIa		B
	Providing sensory and procedural information		Ib	A
	Reframing/cognitive reappraisal	IIa, Va	IIb	B
	Distraction including music	IIa, IIIa, Va	IIb, IIIb	B
	Relaxation, imagery	IIa, IVa	Ib	A
	Biofeedback	IIIa, Va	IIb, IIIb	B
	Psychotherapy and structured support	IIa, Va		B
	Hypnosis	Ia, IIa, Va		A
Physical therapeutic	Superficial heat	IVa, Va		D
	Superficial cold	Va		D
	Massage	IIa, IVa		D
	Active and passive exercise	Va	IIIb, IVb	B
	Immobilization	Va		D
Counterstimulation	Transcutaneous electrical nerve stimulation (TENS)	IVa, Va	Ib	C
	Acupuncture	IVa, Va	IIb, IIIb, IVb, Vb	C

223

A2. Scientific evidence for pain reduction in children

Intervention		Type of evidence		Strength and consistency of evidence
		Cancer patients	Other patients	
Pharmacologic interventions				
Acetaminophen and NSAIDs	Oral (alone)		IIb	D
	Rectal		IIb	B
	Parenteral (ketorolac)		IIb	A
Opioids	Oral	IIIa	IIb	D
	Rectal	—	IIb	D
	Transdermal	IVa	—	D
	Intramuscular (IM)	—	IIb	B
	Subcutaneous (SC)	IVa		D
	Intravenous (IV)	IIa	IIa	A
	PCA (IV and SC)	IIa	IIb	B
	Epidural and intrathecal	IVa	IIb	A
Local anesthetics	Infiltration		IIb	B
	Epidural and intrathecal	Va	IIb	A
	Interpleural		IIb	C
Inhalent analgesia	Nitrous oxide	Va	IIIb	D
Topical anesthetics	Emulsion of local anesthetics (EMLA)	IIa	IIb	A
	Other		IIb	B
Adjuvant analgesic	Psychostimulants	IVa		D
Nonpharmacologic interventions; noninvasive				
Psychosocial	General preparation[1]	IVa	IIb	B
	Providing sensory and procedural information	IIa	IIb	B
	Distraction including music	IIa	IIb	C
	Relaxation		IIb	B
	Biofeedback		IIb	D
	Hypnosis/imagery	IIa	IIb	B
	Parent presence	IIa	IIb	B
Counterstimulation	Transcutaneous electrical nerve stimulation (TENS)	Va		D

[1] Many of these general preparation studies were done in the 1960s to early 1980s. Few of these studies used self-report of pain. Most studies look at behavior, upset, distress, anxiety, and physiologic outcomes.

Type of evidence

I. Meta-analysis of multiple, well-designed controlled studies.

    a.   Studies of patients with cancer.

    b.   Studies of other clinical populations.

II. At least one well-designed experimental study.

    a.   Studies of patients with cancer.

    b.   Studies of other clinical populations.

III. Well-designed, quasiexperimental studies such as nonrandomized controlled, single group pre-post, cohort, time series, or matched case-controlled studies.

    a.   Studies of patients with cancer.

    b.   Studies of other clinical populations.

IV. Well-designed nonexperimental studies, such as comparative and correlational descriptive and case studies.

    a.   Studies of patients with cancer.

    b.   Studies of other clinical populations.

V. Case reports and clinical examples.

    a.   Studies of patients with cancer.

    b.   Studies of other clinical populations.

Strength and consistency of evidence

A. There is evidence of type I or consistent findings from multiple studies of types II, III, or IV.

B. There is evidence of types II, III, or IV, and findings are generally consistent.

C. There is evidence of types II, III, or IV, but findings are inconsistent.

D. There is little or no evidence, or there is type V evidence only.

Panel Consensus—Practice recommended on the basis of opinion of experts in pain management.

Attachment B.

Pain assessment and management instruments

Pain Assessment Instruments for Adults

B1. Brief Pain Inventory (Short Form)

B2. Initial Pain Assessment Tool

B3. Pain Distress Scales

B4. The Memorial Pain Assessment Card

Pain Assessment Instruments for Children

B5. Pain Experience History

B6. Eland Color Scale Figures

B7. Poker Chip Tool Instructions Sheet

B8. Word-Graphic Rating Scale

B9. Pain Affect Faces Scale

Instruments for Pain Management Documentation

B10. Pain Management Log

B11. Flowsheet for Pain Management Documentation

B1. Brief Pain Inventory (Short Form)

Study ID#_____   Hospital#_____

                    Do not write above this line

Date: _____/ _____/ _____

Time:_____

Name:_____ _____ _____
                    Last   First   Middle Initial

1) Throughout our lives, most of us have had pain from time to time (such as minor headaches, sprains, and toothaches). Have you had pain other than these everyday kinds of pain today?   1. Yes   2. No

2) On the diagram, shade in the areas where you feel pain. Put an X on the area that hurts the most.

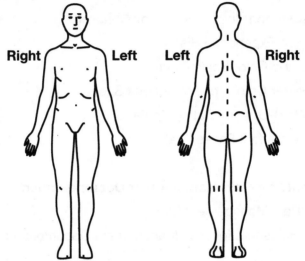

3) Please rate your pain by circling the one number that best describes your pain at its **worst** in the past 24 hours.

0	1	2	3	4	5	6	7	8	9	10
No pain								Pain as bad as you can imagine		

4) Please rate your pain by circling the one number that best describes your pain at its **least** in the past 24 hours.

0	1	2	3	4	5	6	7	8	9	10
No pain								Pain as bad as you can imagine		

5) Please rate your pain by circling the one number that best describes your pain on the **average.**

0	1	2	3	4	5	6	7	8	9	10
No pain								Pain as bad as you can imagine		

6) Please rate your pain by circling the one number that tells how much pain you have **right now.**

0	1	2	3	4	5	6	7	8	9	10
No pain								Pain as bad as you can imagine		

7) What treatments or medications are you receiving for your pain?

_____

8) In the past 24 hours, how much **relief** have pain treatments or medications provided? Please circle the one percentage that most shows how much relief you have received.

0%	10%	20%	30%	40%	50%	60%	70%	80%	90%	100%
No relief									Complete relief	

9) Circle the one number that describes how, during the past 24 hours, **pain has interfered** with your:

A. General activity

0	1	2	3	4	5	6	7	8	9	10
Does not interfere									Completely interferes	

B. Mood

0	1	2	3	4	5	6	7	8	9	10
Does not interfere									Completely interferes	

C. Walking ability

0	1	2	3	4	5	6	7	8	9	10
Does not interfere									Completely interferes	

D. Normal work (includes both work outside the home and housework)

0	1	2	3	4	5	6	7	8	9	10
Does not interfere									Completely interferes	

E. Relations with other people

0	1	2	3	4	5	6	7	8	9	10
Does not interfere									Completely interferes	

F. Sleep

0	1	2	3	4	5	6	7	8	9	10
Does not interfere									Completely interferes	

G. Enjoyment of life

0	1	2	3	4	5	6	7	8	9	10
Does not interfere									Completely interferes	

Source: Pain Research Group, Department of Neurology, University of Wisconsin-Madison. Used with permission. May be duplicated and used in clinical practice.

B2. Initial Pain Assessment Tool

Date_____

Patient's name _____Age _____Room_____

Diagnosis_____Physician_____

Nurse_____

I. Location: Patient or nurse marks drawing.

II. Intensity: Patient rates the pain. Scale used_____

Present:_____

Worst pain gets:_____

Best pain gets:_____

Acceptable level of pain:_____

III. Quality: (Use patient's own words, e.g., prick, ache, burn, throb, pull, sharp)

_____

IV. Onset, duration, variations, rhythms:_____

_____

V. Manner of expressing pain:_____

VI. What relieves the pain?_____

VII. What causes or increases the pain?_____

VIII. Effects of pain: (Note decreased function, decreased quality of life.)

Accompanying symptoms (e.g., nausea) _____

Sleep_____

Appetite_____

Physical activity_____

Relationship with others (e.g., irritability)_____

Emotions (e.g., anger, suicidal, crying)_____

Concentration_____

Other_____

IX. Other comments:_____

_____

X. Plan:_____

_____

Note: May be duplicated and used in clinical practice.
Source: McCaffery and Beebe, 1989. Used with permission.

230

B3. Pain Distress Scales

Simple Descriptive Pain Distress Scale[1]

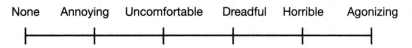

None   Annoying   Uncomfortable   Dreadful   Horrible   Agonizing

0–10 Numeric Pain Distress Scale[1]

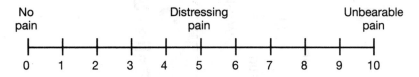

No   Distressing   Unbearable
pain   pain   pain

0   1   2   3   4   5   6   7   8   9   10

Visual Analog Scale (VAS)[2]

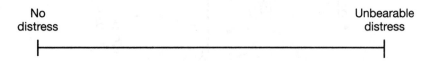

No   Unbearable
distress   distress

[1] If used as a graphic rating scale, a 10 cm baseline is recommended.

[2] A 10-cm baseline is recommended for VAS scales.

Source: Acute Pain Management Guideline Panel, 1992.

B4. Memorial Pain Assessment Card

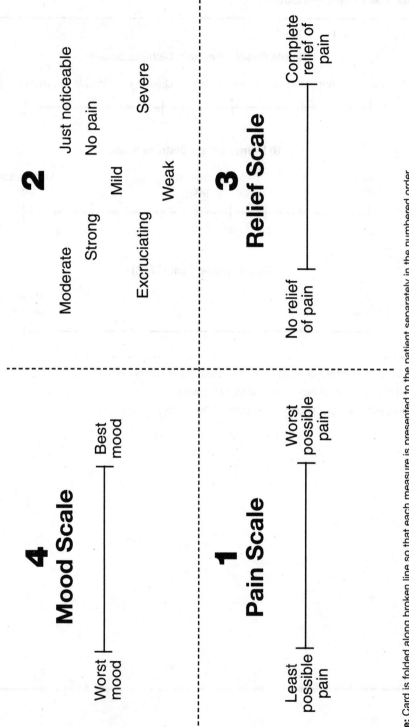

4
Mood Scale

Worst mood ⊢――――――――⊣ Best mood

2

Moderate
Strong
Excruciating
Weak
Mild
Just noticeable
No pain
Severe

1
Pain Scale

Least possible pain ⊢――――――――⊣ Worst possible pain

3
Relief Scale

No relief of pain ⊢――――――――⊣ Complete relief of pain

Note: Card is folded along broken line so that each measure is presented to the patient separately in the numbered order.

Source: Fishman, Pasternak, Wallenstein, et al., 1987. Used with permission.

B5. Pain experience history

Child form	Parent form
Tell me what pain is.	What word(s) does your child use in regard to pain?
Tell me about the hurt you have had before.	Describe the pain experiences your child has had before.
Do you tell others when you hurt? If yes, who?	Does your child tell you or others when he/she is hurting?
What do you do for yourself when you are hurting?	How do you know when your child is in pain?
What do you want others to do for you when you hurt?	How does your child usually react to pain?
What don't you want others to do for you when you hurt?	What do you do for your child when he/she is hurting?
What helps the most to take your hurt away?	What does your child do for him/herself when he/she is hurting?
Is there anything special that you want me to know about you when you hurt? (If yes, have child describe.)	What works best to decrease or take away your child's pain?
	Is there anything special that you would like me to know about your child and pain? (If yes, describe.)

Adapted with permission from Hester and Barcus, 1986.

B6. Eland Color Scale: Directions for Use

After discussing with the child several things that have hurt the child in the past:

1. Present eight crayons or markers to the child. Suggested colors are yellow, orange, red, green, blue, purple, brown, and black.

2. Ask the following questions, and after the child has answered, mark the appropriate square on the tool (e.g., severe pain, worst hurt), and put that color away from the others. For convenience, the word hurt is used here, but whatever term the child uses should be substituted. Ask the child these questions:

   ■ "Of these colors, which color is most like the worst hurt you have ever had (using whatever example the child has given) or the worst hurt anybody could ever have?" Which phrase is chosen will depend on the child's experience and what the child is able to understand. Some children may be able to imagine much worse pain than they have ever had, while other children can only understand what they have experienced. Of course, some children may have experienced the worst pain they can imagine.

   ■ "Which color is almost as much hurt as the worst hurt (or use example given above, if any), but not quite as bad?"

   ■ "Which color is like something that hurts just a little?"

   ■ "Which color is like no hurt at all?"

3. Show the four colors (marked boxes, crayons, or markers) to the child in the order he has chosen them, from the color chosen for the worst hurt to the color chosen for no hurt.

4. Ask the child to color the body outlines where he hurts, using the colors he has chosen to show how much it hurts.

5. When the child finishes, ask the child if this is a picture of how he hurts now or how he hurt earlier. Be specific about what earlier means by relating the time to an event, e.g., at lunch or in the playroom.

Reprinted with permission of J.M. Eland from McCaffery and Beebe, 1989. May be duplicated for use in practice.

Eland Color Scale: Figures

Mark each box with the color the child selects.

No pain No hurt	Mild pain A little hurt	Moderate pain More hurt	Severe pain Worst hurt

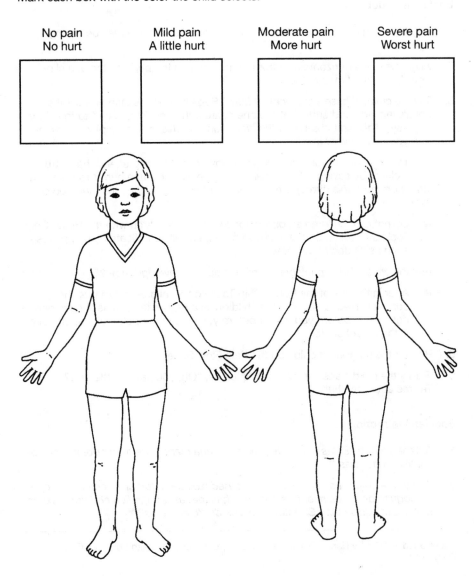

B7. Poker Chip Tool Instruction Sheet[1]

English Instructions:

1. Say to the child: *"I want to talk with you about the hurt you may be having right now."*

2. Align the chips horizontally in front of the child on the bedside table, a clipboard, or other firm surface.

3. Tell the child, *"These are pieces of hurt."* Beginning at the chip nearest the child's left side and ending at the one nearest the right side, point to the chips and say, *"This* (first chip) *is a little bit of hurt and this* (fourth chip) *is the most hurt you could ever have."*

   For a young child or for any child who may not fully comprehend the instructions, clarify by saying, *"That means this* (one) *is just a little hurt, this* (two) *is a little more hurt, this* (three) *is more yet, and this* (four) *is the most hurt you could ever have."*

   - Do not give children an option for zero hurt. Research with the Poker Chip Tool has verified that children without pain will so indicate by responses such as, "I don't have any."

4. Ask the child, *"How many pieces of hurt do you have right now?"*

   - After initial use of the Poker Chip Tool, some children internalize the concept "pieces of hurt." If a child gives a response such as "I have one right now," *before* you ask or *before* you lay out the poker chips, proceed with instruction #5.

5. Record the number of chips on the Pain Flow Sheet.

6. Clarify the child's answer by words such as, "Oh, you have a little hurt? Tell me about the hurt."

Spanish Instructions[2]:

1. Tell the parent: *"Estas fichas de poker son una manera de medir dolor. Usamos cuatro fichas rojas."*

2. Say to the child: *"Las fichas son como pedazos de dolor: una ficha (pedazo) es un poquito de dolor, mientras cuatro fichas (pedazos) significa el dolor máximo que tu puedes sentir. ¿Cuántos pedazos de dolor tienes?"*

---

[1] Developed in 1975 by Nancy O. Hester, University of Colorado Health Sciences Center, Denver, CO.

[2] Spanish instructions by Jordan-Marsh, M., Hall, D., Yoder, L., Watson, R., McFarlane-Sosa, G., & Garcia, M. (1990). The Harbor-UCLA Medical Center Humor Project for Children. Los Angeles: Harbor-UCLA Medical Center.

B8. Word-Graphic Rating Scale

Instructions

"This is a line with words to describe how much pain you may have. This side of the line means no pain and over here the line means worst possible pain." (Point with your finger where "no pain" is, and run your finger along the line to "worst possible pain," as you say it.) *"If you have no pain, you would mark like this."* (Show example.) *"If you have some pain, you would mark somewhere along the line, depending on how much pain you have."* (Show example.) *"The more pain you have, the closer to worst pain you would mark. The worst pain possible is marked like this."* (Show example.)

"Show me how much pain you have right now by marking with a straight, up and down line anywhere along the line to show how much pain you have right now."

No pain	Little pain	Medium pain	Large pain	Worst possible pain

Reprinted with permission from Savedra, Tesler, Holzemer, et al., 1989. [updated 1992]

B9. Pain Affect Faces Scale

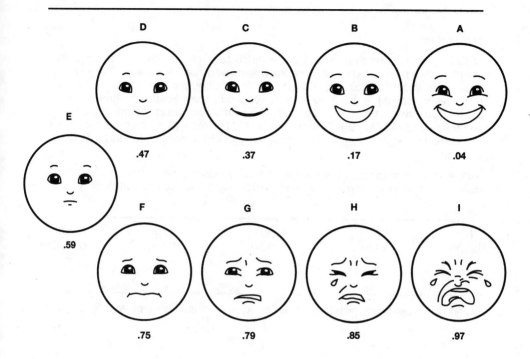

Children are presented with one of three different randomly ordered face sheets. They select the face that best represents how they feel in relation to their pain conditions from "the happiest feeling possible" to the "saddest feeling possible." This figure is actually the scoring card used to quantify children's responses. The numbers represent the magnitude of pain affect (between 0 and 1) shown in each face, based on previous research on children.

Reprinted with permission of McGrath from Patt, 1993.

238

B10. Pain management log

Pain management log for

_____

Please use this pain assessment scale to fill out your pain control log:

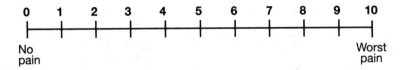

Date	Time	How severe is the pain?	Medicine or non-drug pain control method	How severe is the pain after one hour?	Activity at time of pain

B11. Flowsheet for pain management documentation

Patient_____Date_____

Pain rating scale used [1]_____

Purpose: To evaluate the safety and effectiveness of the analgesic(s)

Analgesics(s) prescribed:_____

Time	Pain rating	Analgesic	R	P	BP	Level of arousal	Other[2]	Plan and comments

Source: McCaffery & Beebe, 1989. Used with permission.

Note: May be duplicated for use in clinical practice.

[1] Pain rating: A number of different scales may be used. Indicate which scale is used and use the same scale each time.

[2] Possibilities for other columns: bowel function, activities, nausea and vomiting, and other pain relief measures. Identify the side effects of greatest concern to patient, family, physician, and nurse.

Attachment C.

Sample relaxation exercises

Exercise 1. Slow rhythmic breathing for relaxation

Exercise 2. Simple touch, massage, or warmth for relaxation

Exercise 3. Peaceful past experience

Exercise 4. Active listening to recorded music

Exercise 1: Slow rhythmic breathing for relaxation

1. Breathe in slowly and deeply.

2. As you breathe out slowly, feel yourself beginning to relax; feel the tension leaving your body.

3. Now breathe in and out slowly and regularly, at whatever rate is comfortable for you. You may wish to try abdominal breathing.

4. To help you focus on your breathing and breathe slowly and rhythmically: (a) breathe in as you say silently to yourself, "in, two, three"; (b) breathe out as you say silently to yourself, "out, two, three."

   or

   Each time you breathe out, say silently to yourself a word such as "peace" or "relax."

5. Do steps 1 through 4 only once or repeat steps 3 and 4 for up to 20 minutes.

6. End with a slow deep breath. As you breathe out say to yourself, "I feel alert and relaxed."

Source: McCaffery and Beebe, 1989. Adapted and reprinted with permission.

Note: May be duplicated for use in clinical practice.

Exercise 2. Simple touch, massage, or warmth for relaxation

Touch and massage are age-old methods of helping others relax. Some examples are:

(1) Brief touch or massage, e.g., handholding or briefly touching or rubbing a person's shoulder.

(2) Warm foot soak in a basin of warm water, or wrap the feet in a warm, wet towel.

(3) Massage (3 to 10 minutes) may consist of whole body or be restricted to back, feet, or hands. If the patient is modest or cannot move or turn easily in bed, consider massage of the hands and feet.

- Use a warm lubricant, e.g., a small bowl of hand lotion may be warmed in the microwave oven, or a bottle of lotion may be warmed by placing it in a sink of hot water for about 10 minutes.

- Massage for relaxation is usually done with smooth, long, slow strokes. (Rapid strokes, circular movements, and squeezing of tissues tend to stimulate circulation and increase arousal.) However, try several degrees of pressure along with different types of massage, e.g., kneading, stroking, and circling. Determine which is preferred.

Especially for the elderly person, a back rub that effectively produces relaxation may consist of no more than 3 minutes of slow, rhythmic stroking (about 60 strokes per minute) on both sides of the spinous process from the crown of the head to the lower back. Continuous hand contact is maintained by starting one hand down the back as the other hand stops at the lower back and is raised. Set aside a regular time for the massage. This gives the patient something to look forward to and depend on.

Source: McCaffery and Beebe, 1989. Adapted and reprinted with permission.
Note: May be duplicated for use in clinical practice.

Exercise 3. Peaceful past experiences

Something may have happened to you a while ago that brought you peace and comfort. You may be able to draw on that past experience to bring you peace or comfort now. Think about these questions:

1. Can you remember any situation, even when you were a child, when you felt calm, peaceful, secure, hopeful, or comfortable?

2. Have you ever daydreamed about something peaceful? What were you thinking of?

3. Do you get a dreamy feeling when you listen to music? Do you have any favorite music?

4. Do you have any favorite poetry that you find uplifting or reassuring?

5. Have you ever been religiously active? Do you have favorite readings, hymns, or prayers? Even if you haven't heard or thought of them for many years, childhood religious experiences may still be very soothing.

Additional points: Very likely some of the things you think of in answer to these questions can be recorded for you, such as your favorite music or a prayer. Then, you can listen to the tape whenever you wish. Or, if your memory is strong, you may simply close your eyes and recall the events or words.

Source: McCaffery and Beebe, 1989. Adapted and reprinted with permission.

Note: May be duplicated for use in clinical practice.

Exercise 4. Active listening to recorded music

1. Obtain the following:
   - ■ A cassette player or tape recorder. (Small, battery-operated ones are more convenient.)
   - ■ Earphone or headset. (This is a more demanding stimulus than a speaker a few feet away, and it avoids disturbing others.)
   - ■ Cassette of music you like. (Most people prefer fast, lively music, but some select relaxing music. Other options are comedy routines, sporting events, old radio shows, or stories.)

2. Mark time to the music, e.g., tap out the rhythm with your finger or nod your head. This helps you concentrate on the music rather than your discomfort.

3. Keep your eyes open and focus steadily on one stationary spot or object. If you wish to close your eyes, picture something about the music.

4. Listen to the music at a comfortable volume. If the discomfort increases, try increasing the volume; decrease the volume when the discomfort decreases.

5. If this is not effective enough, try adding or changing one or more of the following: massage your body in rhythm to the music; try other music; mark time to the music in more than one manner, e.g., tap your foot and finger at the same time.

Additional points: Many patients have found this technique to be helpful. It tends to be very popular, probably because the equipment is usually readily available and is a part of daily life. Other advantages are that it is easy to learn and is not physically or mentally demanding. If you are very tired, you may simply listen to the music and omit marking time or focusing on a spot.

Source: McCaffery and Beebe, 1989. Adapted and reprinted with permission.

Note: May be duplicated for use in clinical practice.

Index

A

Abdominal pain
    causes of, 36
    diagnosis of, 36-37
Ablative surgery
    advantages and disadvantages
        of, 43
    description of, 100-101
    explanation of, 185
Abstinence syndrome, 50-51
Acetaminophen (APAP).
        See also NSAIDs
    advantages and disadvantages
        of, 42, 46
    dosing data for, 48, 49, 55
    recommendations for use of,
        39-41
    scientific evidence for, 222, 224
    used for children, 120-121
    used for elderly patients, 129
    used for neonates and
        infants, 124
    used with opioid analgesics,
        46, 53
Acquired immunodeficiency
        syndrome (AIDS)
    delirium and, 134
    overview of, 139-140
    pain management in patients
        with, 1, 116, 140-141
Acronyms list, 183
Acupuncture
    advantages and disadvantages
        of, 45
    description of, 79-80, 185
    recommendations regarding,
        75, 76, 80
    scientific evidence for, 223
Acute neuralgia, 33-34, 96
Addiction. *See also* Substance
        abusing patients as defined
        in Controlled Substances
        Act, 18
    explanation of, 185
    fear of, 138, 141
    tolerance for opioids vs.,
        39, 50-51, 135, 136
Adjuvant analgesics. *See also* Analgesics;
        Anticonvulsants;
        Antidepressants;
        Bisphosphonates; Calcitonin;
        Corticosteroids; Hydroxyzine;
        Neuroleptic agents; Placebos

    to counteract side effects of
        opioids, 53
    description of, 65, 67-69
    dosing data for, 66
    explanation of, 65, 185
    NSAIDs used with, 46, 53
    recommendations for use of, 39, 40
    scientific evidence for, 222, 224
    used for children, 120-124
Adolescents. *See also* Children
    pain in, 116-117
    patient-controlled analgesia for, 123
AIDS. *See* Acquired immunodeficiency
        syndrome
Alcohol
    drug interactions and, 70
    treatment with intraspinal, 96
American Academy of Pediatrics, 112
American Cancer Society (ACS), 86, 87
American Self-Help Clearinghouse, 87
Amitriptyline
    analgesic effects of, 67-68
    dosing data for, 66, 67
Analgesics. *See also* Adjuvant analgesics;
        Drug therapy; Opioids
    administration methods for, 39,
        62, 126. *See also specific
        methods*
    advantages and disadvantages of, 42
    for postsurgical pain, 35
    principles of use of, 146
    for spinal cord compression pain, 31
    used for children, 120-124
    used for neonates and infants,
        124-125
Anaprox (naproxen sodium), 48
Anterolateral cordotomy, 100-101, 222
Antiarrythmics, 66, 67
Anticonvulsants
    advantages and disadvantages of, 44
    description of, 65, 67
    dosing data for, 66
Antidepressants
    advantages and disadvantages of, 44
    dosing data for, 66
    use of, 67-68, 131
    used for children, 124
    used for elderly patients, 130
Antidiuretic hormone secretion, 65
Antiemetics, 63, 68, 92-93
Antihistamines, 66
Antineoplastic therapies, 70. *See also*
        Chemotherapy
Antiviral therapy, 36

Anxiety, 133-134
Anxiolysis, 185
Anxiolytics
    explanation of, 185
    use of, 68, 110
Arthropan (choline salicylate), 48
Aspirin
    advantages and disadvantages of, 42
    dosing data for, 48, 55
    use of, 41, 46

B
Barbiturates
    long-term use of, 73
    for procedural pain, 111
Behavioral observation
    of children, 119-120
    recommendations regarding, 115, 119
Benzodiazepine, 73, 111, 113
Biofeedback
    advantages and disadvantages of, 44
    explanation of, 185
    scientific evidence for, 223, 224
Biologic therapy, 70
Biopsies, 113
Bisphosphonates, 69
Bone marrow aspiration
    in children, 116
    procedural pain from, 113-114
Bone marrow suppression, 65, 67
Bone metastases
    diagnosis of, 30, 91
    epidural metastases as complication
        of, 30-31
    management of pain due to, 69
    radiation therapy for, 91-93
    recommendations regarding, 89
    to skull, 31, 32
Brachytherapy, 94, 223
Breakthrough pain, 185
Brief Pain Inventory (Short Form),
        26, 228-229
Brompton's cocktail, 73
Bupivacaine, 95
Buprenorphine, 50, 72
Butorphanol
    description of, 50
    risks related to, 72, 73
    use of, 56

C
Caffeine, 53, 61
Calcitonin, 69
Cancer
    in minority patients, 138-139
    prevalence of and mortality from,
        iii, v, 7
    psychiatric problems associated with,
        130-134
Cannabinoids, 72
Carbamazepine
    description of, 65
    dosing data for, 66
    monitoring of patients receiving, 67
Carprofen (Rimadyl), 48
Celiac block, 97, 223
Cervicomedullary junction
        myelotomy, 101
Chemotherapy
    anticonvulsants in patients
        undergoing, 67
    depression and, 131
    description of, 70
    mucositis in patients undergoing, 37
    to treat Kaposi's sarcoma, 140
Cheyne-Stokes respiratory patterns, 129
Children. *See also* Adolescents;
        Infants; Neonates
    assessment of pain management
        strategies for, 127, 128
    drug monitoring in, 124
    drug side effects in, 124
    epidural analgesia for, 126
    HIV infection in, 140-141
    nonpharmacologic methods of pain
        management in, 126, 128
    opioid dosing data for, 52, 54. *See
        also* Opioids
    pain assessment in, 117-120
    pain in, 116-117
    pharmacologic methods of pain
        management in, 120-126, 128, 141
    procedural pain management in,
        107-114
    recommendations regarding
        assessment and treatment of, 115
    scientific evidence for pain reduction
        in, 224, 225
Chloral hydrate, 108
Chlorpromazine, 63, 73, 110
Choline magnesium trisalicylate
        (Trilisate)
    dosing data for, 48

use of, 46-47
used for children, 121
Choline salicylate (Arthropan), 48
Cisplatin, 34
Clinical Practice Guideline for the Management of Cancer Pain
methods used to develop, 20-21
organization of, v, 2-5, 21
purpose and goals of, iii, 1-2
Clonazepam, 65
Clonidine, 51
Cocaine, 72
Codeine
description of, 49-50
dosing data for, 52-55
use of, 41, 45
used for children, 123
withdrawal symptoms from, 51
Coexistent medical conditions
drug therapy and, 70-71
patient screening for, 89, 99
Cognitive reappraisal
explanation of, 185
scientific evidence for, 223
Cognitively impaired patients, 129
Commissural myelotomy, 101, 222
Confusion, 64
Congnitively impaired patients, 115
Conscious sedation
explanation of, 185
management of, 107, 112-113
Constipation
due to opioid use, 40, 61, 62
management of, 61
Controlled Substances Act (CSA), 16, 18
Cordotomy, 100-101, 222
Corticosteroids
advantages and disadvantages of, 44
depression and, 131
description of, 65
dosing data for, 66
for spinal cord compression pain, 31
Counterstimulation
description of, 79-80
explanation of, 185
scientific evidence for, 223, 224
Cryotherapy, 185. *See* Cutaneous stimulation
Cutaneous stimulation
advantages and disadvantages of, 45
description of, 76-78
recommendations regarding, 75, 76
scientific evidence for, 223
used for children, 126

D
Deafferentiation pain, 186
Delirium
effect on pain treatment of, 134
in elderly patients, 129, 134
prevalence of, 130
as side effect of drugs, 131, 134
Dementia
delirium vs., 134
in elderly patients, 129
Demerol. *See* Meperidine
Dependence. *See* Physical dependence
Depression. *See also* Antidepressants
in HIV patients, 140
management of, 131
prevalence of, 9, 130
risk factors for, 131, 132
suicide risk due to, 132, 133
Dexamethasone, 65, 66
Dextroamphetamine
dosing data for, 66, 124
use of, 61
used for children, 124
Dezocine, 50
Diazepam, 111
Didanosine, 140
Diflunisal (Dolobid), 48
Dilaudid. *See* Hydromorphone
Diphenhydramine, 65
Distraction
advantages and disadvantages of, 44
description of, 82, 186
scientific evidence for, 223, 224
use of, 28
used for children, 126
Dolobid (diflunisal), 48
Dolophine. *See* Methadone
Dorsal rhizotomy, 100, 222
Doxepin, 66
Drug therapy. *See also* Adjuvant analgesics; Analgesics; NSAIDs; Opioids; Pain management; *specific drugs*
administration methods for, 39-41, 45, 55-60, 222, 224
discharge planning and, 71
influence of concurrent medical conditions on, 70-71
Medicare reimbursement policies regarding inpatient vs. outpatient, 19
not recommended for cancer pain treatment, 71-73

overview of, 3-4, 40-41
pain assessment following, 28
patient-controlled, 59-60, 123
patient education regarding, 84
for procedural pain, 108, 110-112
recommendations regarding, 39-40
scientific evidence for, 222, 224
to treat cancer, 70
WHO approach to, 12, 14, 41, 45
Dysesthesis, 186

E

Education. *See* Family education;
    Patient education
Eland Color Scale, 234-235
Elderly patients
    drug monitoring in, 47, 111
    drug side effects in, 129-130, 134
    pain assessment for, 115, 129
    pain management in, 129-130
    patient-controlled analgesia used
        by, 130
    prevalence of pain in, 127-129
    recommendations regarding, 115
    rectal opioids in, 56
    renal dysfunction in, 47, 71
Emulsion of local anesthetics
    (EMLA), 111, 224
Endorphins, 102
Epidural
    explanation of, 186
    opioid administration through,
        62, 126
Epidural metastases, 30-31
Equianalgesic, 186
Ethanol, 96
Etidronate, 69
Etodolac (Lodine), 48
Exercises
    description of, 78-79
    recommendations regarding, 75, 76
    for relaxation, 242-245
    scientific evidence for, 223

F

Families
    of children with HIV, 140-141
    pain reduction due to presence
        of, 126, 224
    role in pain assessment and control,
        10-11
    substance abuse within, 141
Family education
    regarding pain and pain
        management, 16

sources of printed information for, 85
Fenoprofen calcium (Nalfon), 48
Fentanyl
    advantages and disadvantages of, 42
    description of, 49-50
    intraspinal, 58
    for procedural pain, 111
    transdermal, 42, 51, 53, 56, 111, 122.
        See also Transdermal opioids
    use of, 45, 53
    used for children, 123
    withdrawal symptoms from, 51
Financial costs, 19-20
Flowchart for Pain Management
    Documentation, 240
Food and Drug Administration
    (FDA), 18

G

Gustave-Roussy Child Pain Scale, 120

H

Hallucinations, 64
Haloperidol, 63
Health care professionals, 17, 18
Health care system, 17
Herpes zoster infection, 96
HIV. *See* Human immunodeficiency
    virus (HIV)
Home care settings, 29
Hormonal therapy, 70, 101
Horner's syndrome, 186
Human immunodeficiency virus
    (HIV), 1, 5, 116, 139-141
Hydrocodone
    description of, 49-50
    dosing data for, 52, 54
    use of, 41, 45
    withdrawal symptoms from, 51
Hydromorphone
    administration methods for, 56, 58
    description of, 49-50
    dosing data for, 52, 54
    use of, 45, 53
    used for children, 123
    withdrawal symptoms from, 51
Hydroxyzine
    advantages and disadvantages of, 44
    to control nausea and vomiting, 63
    description of, 68
    dosing data for, 66
Hypercalcemia
    as complication of bone
        metastases, 30

management of, 69
Hyperpathia, 186
Hypnosis
  advantages and disadvantages of, 45
  description of, 86, 186
  for procedural pain, 113
  scientific evidence for, 223, 224
Hypophysectomy, 101, 222
Hypotension
  opioid antagonists to reverse, 62
  as side effect of methotrimeprazine, 68

I

Iatrogenic, 186
Ibuprofen, 48
Imagery
  advantages and disadvantages of, 44
  description of, 81-82, 186
  scientific evidence for, 223, 224
  used for children, 126
Imipramine, 66
Immobilization
  description of, 79
  recommendations regarding, 75-77
  scientific evidence for, 223
Implanted pumps, 60. *See also*
  Intraspinal administration
Incident pain. *See* Movement-related
  pain
Infants. *See also* Children; Neonates
  analgesics used for, 124-125
  epidural analgesia for, 126
  pain in, 116-117
  recommendations regarding
    assessment and treatment of, 115
  use of pain medication for, 110
Initial Pain Assessment Tool, 26, 230
International Association of
  Laryngectomees, 86
Intramuscular administration, 57, 73
Intraspinal administration
  advantages and disadvantages of,
    60, 102
  dose range for, 58
  indications for, 57-58
  long-term, 58-59
  used for elderly patients, 130
Intrathecal, 186
Intravenous infusion
  advantages and disadvantages of,
    43, 55, 57, 62
  patient-controlled, 59-60
  for procedural pain, 111
  used for children, 122

Intraventricular infusion, 59, 103
Invasive therapies. *See also*
  Neurosurgery; Radiation
  therapy; *specific techniques;*
  Surgery
  overview of, 90
  recommendations regarding, 89-90
  scientific evidence for, 222-223
Isocarboxazid, 70
Isoniazid, 140

K

Ketamine, 110
Ketoprofen (Orudis), 48
Ketorolac tromethamine (Toradol), 48

L

Lancinating, 186
Legislation, 3, 16, 18-19. *See also specific*
  legislation; State legislation
Levo-Dromoran. *See* Levorphanol
Levorphanol
  description of, 49-50
  dosing data for, 52, 54, 64
  side effects of, 134
  use of, 45, 71
  withdrawal symptoms from, 51
Lidocaine
  dosing data for, 66
  used for elderly patients, 129
  used for nerve block, 95
Lodine (Etodolac), 48
Lumbar puncture
  in children, 116
  procedural pain from, 113-114

M

Magnesium salicylate, 48
Massage
  description of, 78
  scientific evidence for, 223
Meclofenamate sodium (Meclomen), 48
Meclomen (meclofenamate sodium), 48
Medicare, 19
Medication. *See* Drug therapy
Mefenamic acid (Ponstel), 48
Memorial Pain Assessment Card, 28, 232
Meperidine
  cautions for use of, 50, 72, 73,
    110, 131
  dosing data for, 52, 54
  hepatic or renal dysfunction and, 71
  for procedural pain, 111
  side effects of, 134

use of, 39, 50
used for children, 123
Methadone
  description of, 49-50
  dosing data for, 52, 54, 64
  hepatic or renal dysfunction and, 71
  maintenance programs using,
    135-137
  side effects of, 65, 134
  use of, 45, 137
  used for children, 123
  used for elderly patients, 129
  withdrawal symptoms from, 51
Methohexital, 110
Methotrimeprazine, 68
Methylphenidate, 61, 63, 66
  dosing data for, 66, 124
  use of, 61, 63
  used for children, 124
Metoclopramide, 53, 63
Mexiletine, 66, 67
Midazolam, 108, 111
Minority patients, 138-139
Mixed opioid agonist-antagonists. *See*
    also Opioids
  cautions for use of, 50
  description of, 49, 50, 186
  recommendations for use of, 39
Monoamine oxidase inhibitors, 70, 131
Morphine
  administration methods for, 56, 58
  for conscious sedation, 112
  description of, 49-50
  dosing data for, 51, 52, 54, 125
  intraspinal, 58
  intraventricular, 59
  methotrimeprazine used with, 68
  for procedural pain, 111
  side effects of, 53, 65, 134
  use of, 45, 136-137
  used for infants and children,
    122, 123, 125, 126
  withdrawal symptoms from, 51
Movement-related pain, 186
Mucositis
  assessment of, 37, 38
  diagnosis of, 37-38
  drug administration during, 55
  explanation of, 187
Music therapy, 187
Myeloma, 33
Myelotomy, 101, 222
Myoclonus, 64, 131
Myofascial pain, 187

N

Nalbuphine
  description of, 50
  risks related to, 72
Nalfon (fenoprofen calcium), 48
Naloxone
  in children, 124
  effects of, 50, 62
  recommendations for use of, 40,
    63, 72
  to reverse hypoventilation, 113
Naltrexone, 72
Naprosyn (naproxen), 48
Naproxen (Naprosyn), 48
Naproxen sodium (Anaprox), 48
Nasal opioids, 56
National Cancer Information Service,
National Cancer Institute Workshop
    on Cancer Pain, 8
National Coalition for Cancer
Survivorship, 86, 87
Nausea, 63
Neonates. *See also* Children; Infants
  analgesics used for, 124-125
  pain in, 116-117
  use of pain medication for, 110
Nerve blocks. *See also* Neurolytic block
  for abdominal pain, 37
  complications from, 97, 98
  description of, 95-98, 186
  for postsurgical pain, 35
  purpose of, 95
Neuopathic pain, 103
Neuraxial opioid infusion, 102
Neuritis, 97
Neuroablation, 100-101
Neuroaugmentation. *See also*
    Transcutaneous electrical ner
    stimulation
  advantages and disadvantages of,
  description of, 102
  scientific evidence for, 223
Neuroleptic agents
  description of, 68
  dosing data for, 66
Neurologic examination, 25, 27
Neurolytic blocks. *See also* Nerve blo
  advantages and disadvantages of
  celiac, 97
  description of, 97-98, 187
  indications for, 97
  recommendations regarding, 89,
  scientific evidence for, 223

Neuropathic pain
  diagnosis of, 33-36
  evaluation for, 26
  explanation of, 187
  management of, 67
Neurosurgery. *See also* Surgery
  to implant drug infusion systems, 102
  neuroablation, 100-101
  neuroaugmentation, 102
  for pain relief, 99-100
  scientific evidence for, 222
Nitrous oxide, 110, 112, 222, 224
Nociceptive pathways
  explanation of, 187
  functioning of, 11-12
NSAIDs. *See also* Acetaminophen;
    specific drugs
  administration methods for, 47
  advantages and disadvantages of,
    42, 46-47
  cost of, 20
  description of, 46-47, 49, 187
  dosing data for, 48, 49
  preparations combining opioids
    with, 52
  scientific evidence for, 222, 224
  use of, 39-41, 49
  used for children, 120-121
  used for elderly patients, 129
  used with opioids and adjuvant
    analgesics, 46, 53
Numorphan. *See* Oxymorphone

O

Opiate receptors
  explanation of, 187
  NSAIDs and, 46
Opioid agonists
  description of, 49, 50, 187
  recommendations for use of, 39, 72
Opioid antagonists, 62, 63, 72
Opioid partial agonist, 49, 50, 187
Opioids. *See also* Drug therapy
  action of endogenous, 12
  adjuvant drugs used with, 53
  administration methods for, 39, 42,
    43, 55-60, 62. *See also specific*
    methods
  advantages and disadvantages of, 42
  cautions regarding use of, 62
  description of, 49-50
  dosing data for, 51-55, 122-123
  fear regarding use of, 16
  following neurolysis, 89

  full, 49-50
  hypersensitivity to, 62
  legal regulation of, 16, 18-19
  long-term use of, 39
  minority patients and, 138
  mixed agonist-antagonist, 49, 50
  NSAIDs used with, 46, 53
  partial agonist, 49, 50
  for procedural pain, 110-113
  recommendations for use of, 39-41, 45
  renal insufficiency and, 71
  scientific evidence for, 222, 224
  side effects of, 40, 50, 61-65, 124
  substance abuse and, 135-138
  tolerance and physical dependence
    on, 39, 50-51, 136
  used for children, 121-124
  used for elderly patients, 129-130
  used for neonates and infants,
    124-125
  withdrawal symptoms from, 51, 96
Orudis (ketoprofen), 48
Oucher, 118
Outpatients
  pain assessment for, 29
  substance abuse by, 137
Oxycodone
  description of, 49-50
  dosing data for, 52, 54
  used for children, 123
Oxymorphone, 52, 56

P

Pain
  as cancer patient problem, iii, v, 1
  discussion of, 7-8, 11-12
  explanation of, 187
  movement-related, 186
  perception of, 12, 128
  procedure-related, 107-114
  quality of life issues related to,
    10-11. *See also* Quality of life
  social spiritual, and physical effects
    of, 11
Pain Affect Faces Scale, 238
Pain assessment
  for children, 117
  of common cancer pain syndromes,
    3, 29-38. *See also specific*
    syndromes
  for elderly patients, 129
  initial, 23-28
  of new pain, 38
  ongoing, 28-29

recommendations regarding, 23, 115, 129
role of family in, 10-11
role of patients in, 3
Pain assessment instruments
for adults, 24, 26-27, 129, 228-232
for children, 118-120, 233-238
for elderly patients, 129
for non-English speaking patients, 29
use of, 24, 26-27
Pain distress scales, 28, 231
Pain Experience History, 233
Pain intensity scales
application of, 26-27
discrepancies in use of, 28
Pain management. *See also*
Drug therapy; Invasive therapies
advantages and disadvantages of various forms of, 42-45
barriers to, 3, 16-19
in children. *See* Children
in cognitively impaired patients, 129
cost and reimbursement for, 19-20
documentation of, 145, 239, 240
in elderly. *See* Elderly patients
flowchart for continuing, 12, 13
in minority patients, 138-139
monitoring quality of, 143-146
in neonates and infants, 110, 115-117, 124-126. *See also* Children
nonpharmacologic, 4
overview of, 12-16
in patients with AIDS, 1, 116, 134, 139-141
pharmacologic, 3-4
priority associated with, 8
for procedural pain, 108-114
role of family in, 10-11
in substance abusing patients, 4-5, 134-138
Pain Management Log, 239
Pain management plans
illustration of, 74
recommendations for use of, 40
requirements for, 71-72
Pain management strategies
assessment in children of, 127, 128
cost involved in various, 20
hierarchy of, 14, 15
Pain syndromes. *See also specific pain syndromes*
assessment of, 3, 29-38
description of common, 29-38

postsurgical, 35, 105
professional awareness of, 23
Palliative therapies. *See also*
Chemotherapy; Radiation therapy; Surgery
explanation of, 187
radiation, 89-94
recommendations regarding, 89
Pamidronate, 69
Pancoast tumor, 187
Panel recommendations
on curricula for health professionals, 3
on invasive therapies, 89-90
on legislation and regulatory policies on use of opioids, 19
overview of, 7
on pain assessment, 23
on pain in special populations, 115-116
on pain management monitoring, 143
on pharmacologic management, 39-40
on physical modalities, 75
on procedural pain, 107
Parents. *See* Families
Pastoral counseling, 45, 75
Patient-controlled analgesia (PCA)
description of, 59-60, 187
recommendations regarding, 62
substance abuse and, 136-137
used by children, 123
used by elderly patients, 130
Patient education
advantages and disadvantages of, 45
goals and benefits of, 83-84
regarding pain and pain management, 16
scientific evidence for, 223
sources of printed information for, 85
Patients. *See also* Children; Infants
drug therapy and concurrent medical conditions in, 70-71
extent of pain in, 7-8
financial resources of, 19-20
lose of control in, 10
minority, 138-139
in outpatient settings, 29, 137
pain assessment in non-English-speaking, 29
pain management plans for discharged, 40, 71-73
pain management problems for, 17
as primary pain assessment source, 3, 24
substance-abusing, 4-5, 115, 134-138

Peer support groups
  advantages and disadvantages of, 45
  description of, 86-87
  methods to locate, 87
  recommendations regarding, 75
Pentazocine
  description of, 50
  hepatic or renal dysfunction and, 71
  risks related to, 72
Pentobarbital, 108
Percutaneous temporary catheter. *See
    also* Intraspinal administration
  use of, 60, 98-99
  used for children, 122
Peripheral neurectomy, 100, 222
Permanent silicone-rubber epidural, 60.
    See also Intraspinal
    administration
Pharmacologic management. *See*
    Drug therapy
Phenol, 96
Phenothiazines
  to counteract side effects of
    opioids, 53
  description of, 68
Phenylzine sulfate, 70
Phenytoin
  description of, 65, 140
  dosing data for, 66
  drug interactions and, 70
  monitoring of patients receiving, 67
Phosphorus-32-orthophosphate, 93
Physical dependence. *See also* Substance
    abusing patients
  explanation of, 188
  on opioids, 50-51, 135
Physical examination, 25, 27
Physical modalities
  explanation of, 76, 188
  forms of, 76-80
  recommendations regarding, 75
  scientific evidence for, 223
Physical therapy, 126
Pituitary, chemical ablation of, 98
Placebos
  knowledge regarding, 12
  recommendations for use of, 40, 69
  response from, 69
Plexopathies
  description of, 93-94
  diagnosis of, 31-33
Poker Chip Tool Instrument Sheet,
    118, 238
Ponstel (mefenamic acid), 48

Positioning, 78-79, 126
Postherpetic neuralgia, 33-36, 96
Postsurgical pain syndromes, 35
Prednisone, 65, 66
Procarbazine, 131-132
Prochlorperazine, 63
Progressive muscle relaxation, 188
Promethazine, 73, 110
Propofol, 110
Propoxyphene, 71
Pruritus, 64, 65
Pseudoaddiction, 135, 188
Psychosocial assessment, 25, 27
Psychosocial interventions
  description of, 80-81, 188
  forms of, 81-87
  recommendations regarding, 75, 81
  scientific evidence for, 223, 224
Psychostimulants, 66, 224
Psychotherapy
  advantages and disadvantages of, 45
  description of, 86
  scientific evidence for, 223
Pyrophosphates, 69

Q
Quality of life, 2, 10-11

R
Radiation therapy
  advantages and disadvantages of, 44
  for bone metastases, 92-93
  cryotherapy following, 77
  indications for palliative, 89
  mucositis in patients receiving, 37-38
  as palliative treatment, 90-91, 94
  for plexopathy, 93-94
  recommendations regarding, 89-91
  scientific evidence for, 223
Radiopharmaceuticals
  for bone metastases, 89, 93
  scientific evidence for, 223
Reach to Recovery, 86
Rectal opioids. *See also* Opioids
  advantages and disadvantages of, 42
  use of, 55-56, 62
Reframing
  advantages and disadvantages of, 44
  description of, 82
  scientific evidence for, 223
Regulatory policies, 3, 16, 18-19
Reimbursement policies, 19-20
Relaxation
  advantages and disadvantages of, 44

description of, 81-82, 188
exercises for, 242-245
scientific evidence for, 223, 224
use of, 28
Renal dysfunction, 47, 71
Respiratory depression
    caused by sedation, 113
    in children, 124
    drug therapy for reversal of
        opioid-induced, 40, 62-64
    effect of, 3-4
    in elderly patients, 129
    management of, 63-64
    in neonates and infants, 125
    opioid plus benzodiazepine
        therapy causing, 111
Rhenium-186, 93
Rhizotomy, 100, 222
Rifampin, 70
Rimadyl (carprofen), 48

S

Salsalate
    use of, 46, 47
    used for children, 121
Samarium-153 phosphonate chelates, 93
Scientific evidence
    for pain reduction in adults,
        222-223, 225
    for pain reduction in children,
        224-225
Scopolamine, 63
Sedation
    conscious, 107, 112-113, 185
    deep, 113
    in elderly patients, 129
    management of, 61, 63
    in neonates and infants, 125
    for procedural pain, 107, 108,
        110-113
    subacute overdose leading to, 64
Seizures, 64
Self-reports. *See also* Pain assessment
    instruments
    for adults, 24, 26-27, 228-232, 239-240
    for children, 118-119, 233-238
Self-statement, 188
Sexual function, 64
Sleep disturbances, 64, 68
Sodium salicylate
    dosing data for, 48
    use of, 46-47
Spinal cord compression
    diagnosis of, 30-31

evaluation for, 26, 29
    management of, 65, 92
Spinal tractotomy, 100-101
State legislation, 18. *See also* Legislation
Strontium-89, 93
Structured support
    advantages and disadvantages of, 45
    scientific evidence for, 223
Subcutaneous implanted injection port,
        60. See also
    Intraspinal administration
Subcutaneous infusion
    advantages and disadvantages of,
        42, 55, 57, 62
    patient-controlled, 59-60
Subcutaneous reservoir, 60. *See also*
    Intraspinal administration
Substance abusing patients
    distinctions among, 135-136
    overview of, 134-135
    pain management in, 4-5, 136-138
    recommendations regarding, 115,
        136, 138
Sufentanil, intraspinal, 58
Suffering, 9-10, 188
Suicide, 132-133, 140
Surgery. *See also* Neurosurgery
    ablative, 43, 99-101, 185
    drug pharmacokinetics following,
        70-71
    pain as consequence of, 105, 222
    pain syndromes following, 35
    principles of, 103
    scientific evidence for, 222

T

Taxol, 34
Teletherapy, 89
TENS, 188
Thermotherapy. *See* Cutaneous
    stimulation
Thiopental, 110
Thought stopping, 113
Tocainide, 66, 67
Tolerance
    explanation of, 188
    for opioids, 50-51, 61, 135, 136
Toradol (ketorolac tromethamine), 48
Transcutaneous electrical nerve
        stimulation (TENS). *See also*
    Neuroaugmentation
    advantages and disadvantages of, 45
    description of, 79
    recommendations regarding, 76, 80

scientific evidence for, 223, 224
 used for children, 126
Transdermal opioids. *See also* Opioids
 advantages and disadvantages of, 42
 for procedural pain, 111
 use of, 51, 53, 56, 62
 used for children, 122
Trazodone, 66
Trilisate. *See* Choline magnesium
 trisalicylate
Tylenol with codeine, 52-55

U

Uniform Controlled Substances Act
 (1990 revision), 18-19
United Ostomy Association, 86
Urinary retention, 65

V

Valproate, 65, 67
Varicella-zoster virus infection, 36
Venipunctures, 116
Vincristine, 34, 140
Vomiting, 63

W

Withdrawal symptoms, 51, 96
Word-Graphic Rating Scale, 237
World Health Organization (WHO)
 analgesic ladder of, 12, 14, 41, 45, 120
 on cancer pain management, 8, 138
 views on use of opioids, 18

Z

Zalcitabine, 140